# Success Stories as Hard Data
## An Introduction to Results Mapping

# PREVENTION IN PRACTICE LIBRARY

SERIES EDITOR

## Thomas P. Gullotta
Child and Family Agency, New London, Connecticut

---

# Success Stories as Hard Data
## An Introduction to Results Mapping

Barry M. Kibel
Pacific Institute for Research and Evaluation
Chapel Hill, North Carolina

Kluwer Academic / Plenum Publishers
New York, Boston, Dordrecht, London, Moscow

Library of Congress Cataloging-in-Publication Data

Kibel, Barry M.
    Success stories as hard data : an introduction to results mapping
    Barry M. Kibel.
        p.    cm. -- (Prevention in practice library)
    Includes bibliographical references and index.
    ISBN 0-306-46071-8. -- ISBN 0-306-46072-6 (pbk.)
    1. Social service--Evaluation.   2. Social policy--Evaluation.
  3. Evaluation research (Social action programs)   I. Title.
  II. Series.
  HV11.K53   1999
  361--dc21                                                    98-31900
                                                                    CIP

ISBN 0-306-46071-8 (Hardbound)
ISBN 0-306-46072-6 (Paperback)

© 1999 Kluwer Academic / Plenum Publishers, New York
233 Spring Street, New York, N.Y. 10013

10 9 8 7 6 5 4 3 2 1

A C.I.P. record for this book is available from the Library of Congress.

Printed in the United States of America

# Foreword

This book offers the first comprehensive introduction to Results Mapping, an innovative approach for assessing the worth of hard-to-evaluate social, health, and education programs. Results Mapping represents a true milestone in program evaluation—a milestone both as methodology for program accountability and as a technique for program improvement. It is relevant across a wide spectrum of public health, social service, and systems-building initiatives. It introduces "new science" into the field of program evaluation. It merges common sense with structured logic. It retains the richness of real world success stories without sacrificing a hard-nosed focus on quantitative data and measurable outcomes.

The contents of this book are directly pertinent for program leadership and staff, for sponsors and funders in the public and private sectors, and for those charged with assessing, documenting and analyzing the effects of program activity. *Success Stories as Hard Data* is designed to be readable, practical, and clear. Its author does not ignore previous scholarly work, but chooses to emphasize real-world applications. For this Dr. Kibel is to be applauded.

Much of traditional evaluation practice owes its evolution to experimental or "demonstration" projects and programs. But such practice too often leads to findings and suggestions that are not very helpful for *ongoing* programs. Surely, more than 99% of all program activity designed to be helpful to citizens is not of the demonstration variety. It is not a question of whether to fund such programs, but rather how to make these funds go farther and accomplish more. And once the question shifts from *Does it work?* to *How can we do it better?*, the nature of evaluation changes.

Results Mapping centers around this latter question. It challenges programs to document and rate their most impactful interventions for, and most helpful support to, those they serve. Indeed, the creative application of this approach and thoughtful attention to the feedback it provides are meant to gently but directly push programs and funders toward:

- discovery of the program's best practices and how best to build on them
- more defensible program and funding strategies
- more realizable program expectations
- more imaginative planning
- more effective use of staff and volunteer power
- more effective collaboration across programs

All these gains help ensure the sponsor's "return on investment."

*Allan Y. Cohen*
*Executive Director*
*Pacific Institute for Research and Evaluation*

# Preface

This book has been written to enable the hard working in community programs to demonstrate their effectiveness to funders and others. It presents a new form of program evaluation called Results Mapping. While based on stories, the approach is not anthropological or merely descriptive. And while the evaluation field has been searching for a creative blend of quantitative and qualitative methods and this new form does this well, we did not set out with the intention of creating a blend. What we were aiming at was building a creative bridge between process and outcome evaluation, something that the evaluation field has also been lacking and demanding.

A brief explanation of "we" is called for here. While I have been the primary architect, chief tester, and driving force behind this new method, I have had—and continue to have—the good fortune to be offered challenging evaluation assignments while being surrounded by the mix of talents required for the approach to reach its potential. The generative force for Results Mapping was first articulated in 1991 by Allan Cohen and myself as we searched for a reasonable way to evaluate a Federal training program that had diverse content and multiple audiences, and was ultimately intended to impact not those attending the training, but others perhaps two or three steps removed from them. Allan is the founder of the Pacific Institute for Research and Evaluation (PIRE) and a leading figure in the field of substance abuse prevention research, evaluation, and practice. Since that time, whenever I have gotten a middle-of-the-night brainstorm *or* stuck, Allan has been the first person I have called for feedback, advice, and guidance. Those who know Allan recognize him as an "open systems" thinker with whom few can compare. Where others find boundaries, Allan always sees new opportunities to merge the known with the unknown.

With Allan's continual support, as well as that of the management team that guides PIRE, I was able to step into that unknown and think what needed to be thought, preach what needed to be preached, and do what needed to be done to give form and substance to a new type of evaluation. We took to the road. The "we" here refers to my wife, Anne Hancock, and me. I hate eating alone in restaurants and I do not look forward to returning to empty hotel rooms after intense days speaking to audiences or consulting on programs and being expected to be both brilliant and useful. Anne gave up her job—admittedly one she was not enamored with—and joined me on these travels, which now have been near continuous for five years. She has made life on the road not only bearable but actually enjoyable. We have eaten well, visited some of America's most interesting urban areas, and met and delighted in the company of many interesting people. Although I have not tested her, in a pinch Anne could probably get up and sell a new audience on Results Mapping. Her support and encouragement are boundless.

New forms of evaluation can take shape only through practice. I agree with Ernie House that evaluation is less "methodology in search of content" than "subject matter in search of appropriate methodology to investigate it" (House, 1994). In this regard, we have had a wealth of subject matter against which to test and improve Results Mapping, and find out where it works and where other methods work better. As I noted earlier, the method was devised as a means for evaluating training programs aimed at intermediaries (i.e., where those receiving the training were not the ones whom the funder *ultimately* wanted to impact). Our client was the Center for Substance Abuse Prevention (CSAP) of the U.S. Department of Health and Human Services. Over a four-year period, we devised multiple means to study the logic of training designs, the quality and fidelity of delivery of training in half-day to week-long sessions, the short-term effects on those who attended the training, the longer-term effects months later as they attempted to integrate the lessons from the training in their workplaces and communities, and the impacts—if any—on those whose behaviors and decisions CSAP was charged with influencing for the better. At that time, we called our approach "open systems evaluation" to acknowledge the influence on these effects and impacts of many factors and forces beyond those within the control of the training programs.

The Department of Mental Health and Addiction Services of the State of Connecticut was our second client. The Department was launching an experiment: providing applied research grants to a select group of agencies to take the best current thinking about what works in prevention and demonstrate that it can work in targeted situations. With foresight, the Department was seeking an evaluation approach that was sufficiently flexible and responsive to match the variety and complexities of the proposed programs. A key member of the advisory group to the Department heard me speak at a conference about our experiences with open systems evaluation and recognized the fit. This led to a contract with the Department and dictated the expansion of the approach beyond assessment of training to areas such as youth development, neighborhood mobilization, institutional impact, and mentoring. Each of these program areas raised tricky evaluation questions; taken together, their evaluation posed a formidable challenge. To help steer us in the right direction, we proposed that a learning community be created. Over the next several years, representatives of the Department, program staff, other prevention specialists from the state, and our evaluation team came together every three to four months to take stock on where the programs were, what the evaluation data were showing, *and* what the evaluation method had become as it went through rapid changes. In hindsight, it had to be changing quickly to guide the thinking of the programs, which themselves were changing as new learning took place. That the Department and the programs put up with the constant changes in assessment method, and actually applauded the breakthroughs that emerged, is a tribute to them as well as a guidepost to the open-mindedness and commitment toward exploration of those who are struggling to turn the art of prevention into a credible and effective discipline.

Until this point, open systems evaluation was exclusively a methodology for the assessment of prevention-focused activity. This changed when I received a call from the United Way & Community Chest of Greater Cincinnati. I had been referred to them by Bill Lofquist, an influential figure in the field of prevention, who had been consulting in that city and recognized a need that I could perhaps fill (Lofquist, 1989; 1996). The Chest had recently launched a multi-year, two-million-dollar annual demonstration. Five community service agencies were each being challenged to merge the funds they received from United Way to operate family resource centers. These centers had the dual purpose of meeting the unique needs of individuals and families in their target communities plus promoting community-based development activities. The family resource center model was founded on the concept of individual and community self-determination. This meant that the center staff were required not only to serve needs and solve problems, but also—in the process—empower their clients to help themselves. United Way was looking for an evaluator with an approach that could gauge the effects of the diversity of services and activity that the centers were generating *and* be credible. What little they heard about the "open systems model" from Bill, and later from reading some articles I had written, suggested to them that we might have the answer.

In those days—less than four years ago, but it feels like ancient history—the open systems evaluation approach we used centered around the creation, in collaboration with the funders and program staff, of customized scoring systems for gauging the relative value of program activities. These scores were then used to assign worth to the results of a program's activities. To rate prevention activities, for example, a raw score of 1 might be assigned to the messages received through the media, a raw score of 2 for exposure to a motivational speaker, and a raw score of 3 for skills received through training. To capture the work of the family resource centers, special codes with point values were devised for the broad array of emergency services, social services, prevention activities, and community development functions that engaged their staffs. While all of us involved in the process—

United Way staff, family resource center staffs, agency heads, and myself—recognized that we had moved into unfamiliar territory, the promise of a fresh approach to the evaluation of social and community services intrigued enough of us to allow experimentation in an area where a lot of money was at stake.

The family resource center evaluation is now in its fourth year. We have moved from the open systems model to Results Mapping, making this transition between years two and three. This was the first application of Results Mapping in which annual funding decisions are being linked to the evaluation results. The collaborative spirit that has permeated the process, plus the flexibility and thoughtfulness of the United Way and family resource center staffs, have allowed the evaluation to be reshaped within this high-stakes environment to best meet the needs of all stakeholders.

Cincinnati is one of those cities where everyone seems to know one another. Within weeks of setting out on this new evaluation path, the phone started ringing. Other agencies in the city with United Way connections had heard about the open systems approach and wanted to see if it would fit their evaluation needs. During the next year, I had the opportunity to provide consulting and set up mini-evaluations to address such diverse program areas as senior centers, family preservation, school truancy, parent education, and foster care. The county (Hamilton) had also recently launched an experiment of its own: providing intensive care management services through public resources to nearly 300 youth for whom the county was spending a large share of its service dollars. These youth ranged in age from 6 to 21 and included those with long criminal histories, those with substance abuse problems, those with multiple service needs, and some with mental retardation and/or developmental disabilities. I was asked to modify the open systems model to permit ongoing estimation of the benefits to these youth and their families of this public managed care approach. Soon after launching this evaluation, we were successful in winning a large, multi-year grant from the Substance Abuse and Mental Health Services Administration to conduct a multi-modal evaluation of the program. This is allowing us to contrast more traditional outcome assessments with those derived through Results Mapping.

To paraphrase the words of wise King Solomon, any time you think that you are out there doing something new and different, you will soon discover others who have thought of it, done it, and even called it the same thing you named it. So it was with "open systems evaluation." As word of our work began to spread, friends and colleagues began sending me articles and papers, some decades old, that discussed evaluation in much the same terms as we now did and even sometimes using the term "open systems evaluation." We were obviously not the first to recognize the complexity of social programs and the messiness of the environments in which they operate. While most evaluators had taken the more traditional path of standing back and employing quasi-experimental paradigms—in some cases, very creatively (Trochim, 1986)—to investigate the effects and impacts of complex programs, some had jumped into the flow of participatory consciousness and were pushing the boundaries of the field into empowerment evaluation (Fetterman, Kaftarian, & Wandersman, 1996) and common-sense evaluation (Morrell, 1979). In the latter category, I was particularly impressed with a short book by Michael Scriven, which offered 31 practical insights into program evaluation (Scriven, 1993).

Among my favorites were these insights, which I still hold dear:

#2. Program evaluation is *not* applied social science.
#4. Side effects are often the main point.
#8. Pure outcome evaluation usually yields too little too late, and pure process evaluation is usually invalid or premature.
#11. Rich description is not an approach to program evaluation but a retreat from it.
#19. "Pulling it all together" is where most evaluations fall apart.
#21. Validity and credibility do not ensure utility.

There remained enough differences between our work and that of the other open systems evaluators that I felt it was important to set us apart. This led, in late 1995, to a search for a unique name for what had evolved into a very specific method. The name selected was Results Mapping.

I had spent the 1970s living in Jerusalem and teaching at the Hebrew University. During that period, I became familiar with some interesting work of the measurement theorist Louis Guttman. He had devised an original way of capturing complicated data sets that did not easily collapse to numbers. These data were arrayed in structured formats, akin to fill-in-the-blank sentences, which he called "mapping sentences." The theory and statistics associated with Guttman's work (referred to as facet theory) were well beyond my levels of interest and mathematical reasoning (Shye, Elizur, & Hoffman, 1994). However, I was intrigued by the elegance of the concept of capturing data through formalized sentences. Twenty years later, when I was engaged in analyzing the complex data set from the training study discussed earlier, I remembered Guttman's mapping sentences. As it turned out, the approach did not fit as well as I hoped it might. But after some manipulations coupled with a few additions of my own making, the "results map" took shape. It has been the focus of my work in evaluation ever since.

The past three years on the lecture circuit, coupled with several dozen small and medium-sized consulting contracts, have provided a priceless opportunity to refine the approach. The rules and conventions of Results Mapping have undergone multiple adjustments and outright changes during these three years as the methodology has evolved and matured. We have not been whimsical. Our aim throughout has been to increase the method's reliability. This twofold aim has involved (1) creating and applying mapping rules that translate narrative accounts of a program's best work into structured forms (i.e., mapped stories) without distortion, while (2) devising and applying coding and scoring conventions to these mapped stories that lead to fair ratings and accurate measures of program contributions toward long-term client success. The originality and complexity of the most outstanding work of programs kept driving us back to the drawing board to determine how best to capture their achievements using maps and scores. Of late, the changes we have made in the methodology have been relatively modest even as the volume of stories we have reviewed has increased manyfold. This provides some measure of hope that only modest tweaking may be needed in the months ahead and that this document will continue to serve as the definitive textbook for the approach.

Returning to the topic of "we," there are a few additional persons who need to be singled out here. During the open systems evaluation era (roughly 1991–1996), in addition to Allan Cohen, I benefited from feedback from two forward-thinking Federal employees, Len Epstein and Steve Seitz, who were not afraid to demand nonconventional evaluations for the innovative training programs they helped oversee at CSAP. Len encouraged us to assemble and pay attention to advice from a formidable advisory group that included some outstanding evaluators: Larry Green, Paul Florin, Abe Wandersman, Jean Ann Linney, and Ron Braithwaite.

Our own team at PIRE included some original thinkers about evaluation, most notably Judith Ottoson, Margo Hall, and Tara Kelley-Baker. Throughout this period and continuing into the Results Mapping era (1996–1998), I have frequently traded ideas and *Aha!* moments with my sidekick, Will Miner. During the latter era, two bright new Ph.D.s joined with me in forming PIRE's Results Mapping Laboratory in Chapel Hill and pushing the approach to new heights. Al Stein-Seroussi and Dave Currey are continually asking the hard questions, building bridges to other complementary approaches, and providing real-time support for our growing client base. The glue that holds the whole thing together is provided by Janet Jester, our office manager in Chapel Hill. Those who have benefitted from the multiple gifts of a great-natured, super-efficient, and ever-helpful support person know just how critical someone like Janet is to the success of a fledgling operation.

In addition to reminding us that "there is nothing new under the sun," King Solomon also pointed out that "for all things, there is a season." The timing could not be better for the emergence of Results Mapping. We have entered the era of outcome-based accountability. Funders of all types—public and private, Federal to local—are interested in outcomes, not processes. They want evidence that programs they fund are making significant contributions and catalyzing changes, for the better, in the lives of their clients. And, further, they want this evidence to be concrete and valid (not "anecdotal").

The programs we have been asked to evaluate do not fit a mold. They do not produce the same outcome, nor even a small set of outcomes, again and again. In fact, they are *not* outcome *producers*. They offer no magic bullets or panaceas for the problems besetting individuals, families, neighborhoods, communities, and systems. They can, however, be exceedingly helpful to those they serve. At their best, they focus on client assets, not deficits. They raise spirits. They offer hope. They untangle knots. They set people on the path to new life possibilities. They help make difficult outcomes possible.

These programs need to be evaluated on *their* terms.

One final note: Each chapter of the book ends with a short quiz. The questions were not designed to test memory recall. Thus, the answers will not be found by looking back into the chapter. The questions are of two types: some are meant to be thought provoking and stimulate a deeper appreciation of the approach; others provide practice in applying the rules and conventions of Results Mapping. The quizzes can be skipped without fear of missing essential information. My answers to the questions appear in Appendix A. In some cases, they are not the only answers possible.

# Contents

## Part I  Theory

## Part II  Practice

# I

# Theory

# A Different Kind of Evaluation

*Whatever else evaluation may be, it must concern itself with outcome, i.e., with the influence of a social program on its clients and/or its societal context (Morell, 1979, p. 1)*

Many health and social programs and virtually all community development efforts share a common dilemma. The best of what they do—the transformations and healing they help catalyze, as well as their short-term contributions to longer-term outcomes—cannot be easily measured. This makes it difficult to demonstrate their successes and full worth to funders, Boards, and others.

The best illustration of a program's work is frequently found in stories that relate its most dramatic successes with clients. These are the stories that program staff present to their Boards, share at conferences, or pull out when soliciting funds, and are the ones that sometimes reach the media. But funders and others who seek proof of program benefits are suspicious of such stories, and with good reason. A few anecdotes about remarkable client turnarounds generally represent the exceptions to the rule and do not offer a true picture of what a program does on a day-to-day basis with most of its clients. Faced with a choice between receiving colorful narratives on a select few clients or colorless data on all or most program activities, funders have invariably opted for the latter. "Show us the numbers!"

Toward this end, a program focused on healing or client transformations will typically report body counts of those it has served, results from client satisfaction surveys, and an assortment of numeric measures of client or community outcomes, while engaging in a *qualitatively different* enterprise with its clients than these quantitative indicators reveal. Such a program will likely deliver more than the routine services indicated by such counts; it will work *with* its clients in unique and complex ways, frequently beyond standard work hours and over extended periods, helping them to gain control over difficult life situations and

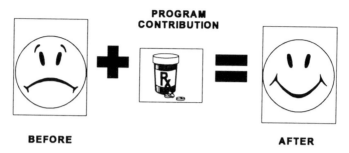

Figure 1.1. Easy attribution. Only these pills seem to explain why the client felt better.

move beyond current crises. In place of remedies for all that ails its clients, the program will offer the resources and support necessary for its clients to exercise increased self-determination—hopefully leading, over time, to improved health and life quality.

Program staff are the first to admit that the numeric data they provide just skim the surface of program activity and relate little about the wondrous transformations that may have occurred with *specific* clients or target populations. They recognize that the parts of stories that give goosebumps and show the program in its best light, as well as key descriptive data, are missing from their reports.

The program's numbers tell little about the clients who have progressed beyond dependency on the service delivery system to heal themselves and become healing supports to others. They also reveal little regarding the innovative work of staff with difficult-to-serve clients, even when no dramatic outcomes have yet occurred; or of pioneering efforts of the program to partner with other service providers and community agents to serve clients who heretofore were not reached or who could not afford the type and range of services they desperately needed.

A program is ultimately only as good as the outcomes it generates. Nothing could be more straightforward. The purpose of evaluation, above all else, is to document what these outcomes are—with clarity and integrity.

And it is easy to be clear about the case illustrated in Figure 1.1. The outcome is a happy client. Before ingesting the pills, the client was not happy. The pills seemed to have done the trick. The program that provided the pills is credited with the outcome.

But what about the next case (Figure 1.2)? Here we have a client who has received counseling from a program. In conducting a follow-up interview with the client, the program's evaluator discovered that he had won the lottery. Now what was responsible for the happiness, the counseling or the lottery win, or both? And how much is each responsible? If the winning ticket was worth only $10, we might still attribute the change to the counseling and give the program full credit for the

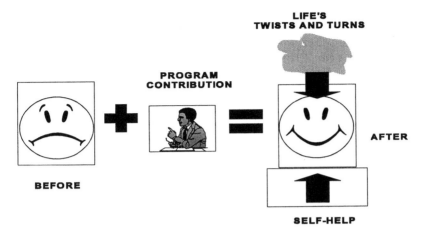

Figure 1.2. Tricky attribution. Life's twists and turns, as well as the growth of the client, could account for why the client felt better.

outcome. However, if this was a $15 million jackpot, then one might wonder if the counseling mattered all that much.

And there may be yet another factor at work here. Forget the lottery. By the time the program's evaluator gets to interview the client, he has changed. He is a happier person. He just decided to grow up and be happy. When we ask what caused the change, he can't say. He just got tired of being grumpy. It wasn't getting him anywhere. He wasn't moving on with his life. He felt the need to change...and did.

But let's go further. Recognizing, as in the above example, that its clients may likely be influenced by life's twists and turns *and* by self-motivated growth, the program chooses to work with these realities and not worry about the inability to attribute credit. After all, this is its evaluator's problem, not its own. The program does not represent itself as being in the fix-it business (as might a program whose work looks like Figure 1.1). Instead it provides a set of customized services to each of its clients, including in some cases pills or counseling, that as an integrated package are designed to bring the client closer to the desired outcome. And furthermore, it takes a long view. It aims to contribute not only to short-term changes in the client but also to downstream outcomes—maybe months or even years into the future. To make this possible, it teams up with other service providers in the community to offer its clients a full range of options, well beyond what it can provide alone. (Its work with one such client is portrayed in Figure 1.3.)

This is not just a made-up argument for the sake of argument. The most outstanding work of many social and health programs looks more like Figure 1.3 than

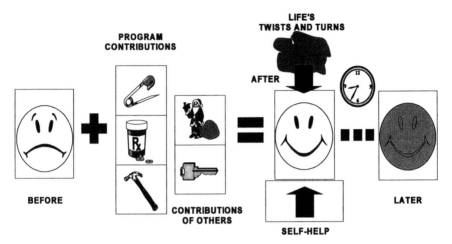

Figure 1.3. Complex attribution. The client has been influenced by several program services, by the services of others to whom the client has been referred by the program, by life's twists and turns, and especially through personal growth processes. Further, as time passes, the client has retained these outcomes.

like either Figures 1.1 or 1.2. Is it any wonder that they get nervous when funders start demanding, as conditions for funding, that they demonstrate that their clients are achieving outcomes using the same logic and reporting format as might a program in the fix-it business?

And prevention programs are in an even worse predicament because they are specifically charged with helping produce the longer-term outcomes. They have to deal not only with the complexities associated with contributing to short-term change, but also with the effects of time (which are symbolized in Figure 1.3 by the clock). Over time, the short-term gains catalyzed by the program can diminish or disappear—as old habits kick in and new factors appear and begin to influence the client. A prevention program that, for example, provides an after-school program for sixth graders *and* expects to see them successfully completing high school—drug-free, child-free, and with a lifelong lust for learning—may be expecting too much.

To complete the set, allow me to introduce one last figure (Figure 1.4) that illustrates the increased difficulty of evaluating programs aimed at intermediaries.

Figure 1.4 resembles Figure 1.3, but has a further complication. Here the program has the opportunity to influence the short-term and longer-term outcomes of client A, who, in turn, is responsible for influencing the outcomes for person(s) B. For example, client A may be a group of parents who have poor academic skills but desire to support the education of their young children (B). The role of the pro-

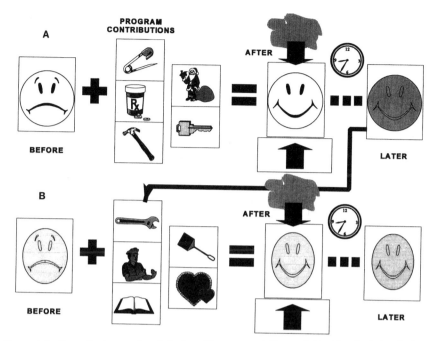

Figure 1.4. Exceedingly complex attribution. The program influenced client A, who in turn had responsibility for influencing A's client B. Lots of services, direct and indirect, as well as lots of growth and time, stand between the program and these ultimate outcomes for B.

gram is to strengthen these skills so that the parents, in turn, can read to their children, help with homework, and encourage their intellectual development. Or, to use a community development example, a program may be charged with training and providing technical assistance to a community coalition attempting to reduce problem drinking in its city. The coalition (client A), in turn, will be attempting to influence the behaviors of those engaged in this problem drinking (B). It was this type of evaluation challenge, as was discussed briefly in the opening chapter, that prompted us to develop what has evolved into Results Mapping. Our charge was not only to assess the short-term effects and longer-term outcomes on a large population of trainees (client A), but also to determine how what they learned translated to outcomes for the individuals, groups, neighborhoods, and whole communities (B) that they, in turn, served.

With this broad picture in mind, let's start again at the beginning. The types of programs best positioned to demonstrate that they are outcome producers are what I refer to as "fix it/cure it" programs. In the extreme case, one such program will offer a single intervention (e.g., a flu shot or brief intervention) in expectation of some favorable future outcome (e.g., continued or enhanced health). Clients are passive recipients of the program's service. Since each client gets the same service with expectations of a similar result, the program's body counts and success rates alone provide good and near complete proof of program performance. A fix it/cure it program of this type would not typically tell client stories; however, should it agree to partake in storytelling, one such anecdote might read:

> A female came into the clinic, received the standard service, and—through follow up by telephone—was found to have been helped (i.e., the problem that prompted the visit has been resolved).

If asked for a second story, it would be virtually identical with the first. In fact, all stories would be virtually identical. And that story line would not likely generate many goose bumps with funders, Board members, or others. Numbers work best here.

Contrast the relative simplicity of that story with the one following from a residential center for homeless youth:

> Mary is now 19 years old and about to enter the local university on a full scholarship. When she was referred to our program three years ago, her future looked bleak. She had quit school, was hanging out on the streets, and was drinking heavily. She had attempted suicide three times, the last resulting in her placement in our residential center. Mary was not an ideal client. She disappeared on four separate occasions, the longest period lasting six months, from which she returned pregnant. After that, she agreed to abide by our rules and norms, participated actively in group counseling, bonded with one of our staff, gave up drinking and smoking, delivered a healthy baby, completed her high school education, got a job, moved into her own apartment, and competed successfully for the scholarship.

With a story like Mary's, we have moved from the realm of simple attribution into the realm of complex attribution. Linking services to outcomes is no longer an automatic exercise.

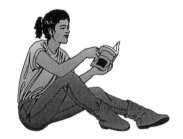

The next chart (Figure 1-5) contrasts the differences, at the extreme, between these two realms.

There is not a sharp boundary between the two realms, but rather a transition to ever-

|  | Realm of simple attribution |  | Realm of complex attribution |
|---|---|---|---|
| Number of services | one | ➡ | multiple |
| Variation in services | none | ➡ | wide |
| Influence of "outside factors" | weak | ➡ | strong |
| Distance from services to outcomes | short | ➡ | long |
| Number of outcomes | one | ➡ | multiple |
| Diversity of outcomes | none | ➡ | rich |
| Role for client | passive | ➡ | active |

Figure 1.5. Contrast between the realms of simple and complex attribution. In the simple extreme, there is a single service virtually *causing* a single outcome. In the complex extreme, there are multiple services *associated with* multiple outcomes.

increasing complexity. With a simple story, a program provides a single service to a client in hopes of causing a single outcome in the not-too-distant future. As programs provide more and varied services, as well as network with other agencies to support client needs, stories become more complex and thus also does attribution. The program's multiple efforts each *contribute* in varying degrees toward the attainment by the client of a range of diverse outcomes. Some of these occur soon after services are delivered, while others may not occur until months or years following the services.

The logic underlying simple attribution is *causal*. The contention is that the single program service is responsible for the single outcome; stated in brief, it has caused it. Other possible causes of that outcome are considered either nonexistent or insignificant. In contrast, the logic underlying complex attribution is *synchronistic*. Events are linked in time and space through connections and associations that overlap and influence one another. Outside factors beyond the reach of the program may influence outcomes as much or more than the program's services. Further, in some cases, the client may be as likely to influence the program and the services it provides as the program is to influence the client. And, even more dramatic, the client may heal or grow from within.

In fact, the essential feature of complex systems—be these molecules, cellular structures, persons, families, teams, neighborhoods, communities, organizations, or institutions—is that, in them, new and previously undetected and unpredicted properties can and do *emerge* (Waldrop, 1992). These properties emerge when the proper conditions are ripe for their emergence. It is less an issue of time passage than of readiness for change. Modern physicists call this the generative order of space–time (Bohm & Peat, 1987).

One day, my daughter is a young girl; the next, she is suddenly a woman. What happened during the night to make the difference? For years, America was waging the cold war against the Russians. Suddenly, it was over. We did not "nuke" the Russians into submission. What happened was that our world transformed, emerging with new properties and possibilities. One can look for causes in the global economy, the information revolution, the inability of the Russians to match our defense spending, the mounting pressures of the culturally and nationally diverse elements of the Soviet system, and the incompatibility of a "closed political-social system" within an open, dynamic, modern world society. But suddenly, seemingly overnight, there was and remains a post-cold war reality.

Almost a century ago (December 20, 1900), a major revolution was launched in the field of physics. In a presentation to a group of distinguished scientists, Max Planck introduced the world to a new concept, the *quantum* of energy. He is reported to have employed the following metaphor to explain the concept:

> Imagine, in the world as you know it, that I throw a rock into a still pond. Two things would happen. First, the rock would sink to the bottom of the pond. Second, there would be a ripple effect across the pond. Now let us enter a different world, which we will call the world of quantum mechanics. I throw a rock into a still pond. But only one thing happens. The rock sinks to the bottom of the pond. There is no ripple effect. This surprises me. So, I find a large boulder and heave it into the pond. The boulder sinks to the bottom, but still there is no ripple effect.
>
> As I sit at the edge of the pond staring out at it in amazement, a young child skips by. She stops and throws a small pebble into the pond. Suddenly the pond erupts and produces the combined ripple effects of all the rocks, boulders, and pebbles that have ever been thrown into it. Potential energy has been activated. It appears to take a critical amount of energy—a quantum's worth—for certain types of changes to occur. Until that level is reached, the potential for change builds but is not actualized. However, the instant that the critical threshold is crossed, fundamental change must occur. There is a new kind of lawfulness at work here.

When programs engage their clients in healing and transformation, the energies and dynamics at play are more like those associated with the quantum pond than those of the pond of immediate cause and effect. In the quantum physics example, the pond is storing energy, while in the case of a client what is being accumulated is "readiness to change." Programs can add to this readiness or, with bad practice, decrease client readiness (akin to removing a rock and its energy from the pond). In the causal realm (what I call the realm of simple attribution), program success is linked directly to outcomes produced (i.e., to the ripple effects). In the quantum realm (the realm of complex attribution), success is linked to building readiness (i.e., to the boulders, rocks, and pebbles added to the pond).

Different conclusions can be drawn regarding program contribution depending on the realm within which one views the program. To illustrate:

> A program had two new clients whose histories and problems appeared similar. At the initial meeting with the first client, the staff provided a routine intervention and the client achieved a dramatic breakthrough. Her life turned around and she moved on to a happy and healthy life filled with adventures and successes.

The program threw a pebble or small rock into the pond and was rewarded with an immediate and dramatic ripple effect. All that was apparently needed for her to cross the threshold was that small dose of added readiness triggered by the routine intervention.

> Success with the second individual proved far more elusive. Months of services, including creative use of techniques that had earned national recognition, yielded only modest progress. There were advances, followed by relapses, and long periods with no movement at all. The client ultimately dropped out of the program having failed to overcome her problems. Two years later, this second client was talking with a friend at a restaurant. Suddenly, all the pieces of her life came together. She erupted in laughter. Starting that night, she began making major changes in her life and, like the first client, went on to a life filled with successes.

The program had heaved boulders, rocks, and pebbles into the pond, but no ripples occurred. The pond was perhaps brought to the brink of readiness, but it took at least one additional pebble thrown several years later to trigger the ripples.

This raises an interesting question. Did the program succeed with the first client and fail with the second? It depends on how one looks at things:

☺☹ If the measure of success is the *level of outcome* reached while the client is in the program or even within a year of leaving the program, then the first case was more successful than the second.

☺☹ If the measure of success is *reaching a major milestone* while a client is in the program, the first case succeeded and the second case failed.

☹☺ If the measure of success is *total contributions* made through the program toward a client's healing, then the second case was more successful.

There are programs whose essential challenge is to fix and cure. There are other programs whose essential challenge is to help their clients to grow and/or heal. These two types of programs operate differently. They need to be evaluated differently.

For both types of programs, outcomes may result. For the first type, the test of success is the ability to produce these outcomes. For the second type, the test of success is the ability to contribute to changes in the behaviors and status of their clients. As these changes occur, outcomes should result. But they are not produced *by* the program and it is misleading and a disservice to these programs to think solely or primarily in these terms.

# QUIZ 1

1.1. As commonly used, what are the differences between program inputs, outputs, outcomes, impacts, and results?

1.2. When does it make sense to invest evaluation dollars in outcome measurement? When does it make sense to invest evaluation dollars in community impact measurement? And when would it make more sense to invest these dollars in an approach such as Results Mapping?

1.3. What makes prevention programs more difficult to evaluate than treatment programs? What is the "bottom line" against which prevention programs ought to be judged?

# 2

# Why Success Stories?

*Information in chemical, nutritional, or language form is es-
sential to growth at any level. In the interactive processes of
growth, sharing of information provides the possibilities of
growth. The more appropriate the available information is,
the more growth can occur (Land, 1973, p. 14).*

Effective program evaluation is information-rich. The primary use of this information is to assure the program's supporters that desirable outcomes are happen-
ing through the actions of the program *and* in sufficient quantity *and* with enough
quality. In addition, the information provided should validate, if not celebrate, the
hard and sometimes outstanding work of program staff in making these outcomes
more likely. Further, the information should detect program shortfalls that ought
to be corrected and pinpoint program strengths and emerging opportunities that
can be exploited to increase program contributions toward these outcomes.

For "fix it/cure it" programs, the best form of information is numeric. Numbers are relatively easy to gather, combine, analyze, and use to draw conclusions
regarding program performance. Further, the link between services and outcomes
(the zone where stories might best be told) is simple, undramatic, and short.

For programs engaged in healing, transformation, and prevention, the best
source and form of information are client stories. It is through these stories that we
discover how program staff interact with clients, with other service providers, and
with family and friends of their clients, to contribute to outcomes; and how the clients, themselves, grow and change in response to program inputs and other forces
and factors in their lives. There is a richness here that numbers alone cannot capture. It is only for a story not worth telling, due to its inherent simplicity, that numbers will suffice.

13

There are, however, some inherent difficulties in relying on stories as the principal source of program evaluation information. First among these is the time and effort it takes to capture a story. Most programs do not spend much time following up with their clients to find out what happened to them after interacting with the program. While

| Obstacles to the Use of Stories as Evaluation Data |
| --- |
| 1. Time and effort |
| 2. Storytelling technique |
| 3. Getting the story straight |
| 4. Consistency across stories |
| 5. Aggregating the information |

there has been a dramatic shift from process toward outcome measurement across the nation, adequate compensation for time needed to determine what these outcomes have been has not been forthcoming. Somehow, programs are expected to measure their outcomes but with little or no new money or staff time devoted to this venture. So most programs simply muddle through, capturing outcomes in an ad hoc manner to meet funder requirements or to demonstrate that their promised productivity has been reached or surpassed. Consequently, the stories they can relate about their work with clients are incomplete. This is unfortunate. A lot of learning can occur if time is taken to find out what really worked and what worked less well or not at all in the months that followed the interaction period. Did short-term gains persist? Did what looked like a failure actually turn into a success?

A second difficulty is more fundamental. Most people lack the training and skills needed to be good storytellers for evaluation purposes. They tend to ramble, skip key points while dwelling on incidentals, and get the logic and order of the story mixed up. Related to this is a third difficulty. The person telling the story—most often the program staffer who has had most contact with the client featured in that story—may not know the whole story. Other staff may have been involved at the beginning who have moved on to other jobs. Further, the client will likely have details or know of factors influencing the outcomes that no one in the program has heard about.

Even when the stories are complete and accurate, the styles of relating them will vary greatly across storytellers. This is a fourth difficulty. And finally, assuming we can achieve accuracy, completeness, and consistency in a data base of stories, how can the varied information within these stories be combined to draw findings and conclusions useful to funders, program staff, and others?

These are some of the major issues that we have been struggling with in the development of Results Mapping as an alternative or complementary form of evaluation for programs engaged in healing, transformation, and prevention. And, I am pleased to report, we have arrived at reasonable solutions to each of them. The remaining materials in this book present and illustrate these solutions. In this chapter, as a way of introducing the approach, partial answers will be offered to each difficulty listed above.

Before proceeding with these answers, however, I should first explain what we mean by a "story." The following is a narrative account of a story (written in September 1997) included in an evaluation of a senior center.[1]

> Frances is a 78-year-old currently residing in Cincinnati. She moved here eight months ago from Florida, after the death of her husband, to live with her daughter. She required some surgery in March and was homebound for four weeks. During that time, she received warm lunches through the meals-on-wheels program operated by our senior center. This was her first contact in Cincinnati with adults her own age. The volunteer who delivered the meals (John F.) encouraged her to visit the center after she got well. She arrived one day, stayed a few hours then left. A week later she was back, and remained most of the day. She has been a regular ever since. For the past two months, she has been volunteering in the kitchen helping to prepare the meals we deliver.

Note that this is not a life history of Frances. The narrative focuses on her relationship with the program, a senior center in Cincinnati. Included is the first contact with the program from which she benefitted, followed by other interactions leading to contributions to her life. Also included are milestones reached by her and actions she has taken to benefit others (that are directly or indirectly traceable back to the program encounters). This narrative would be translated into a set of six results maps, each map documenting some major program action or related activity key to Frances' growth or well-being.

All maps in Results Mapping have the same basic structure:

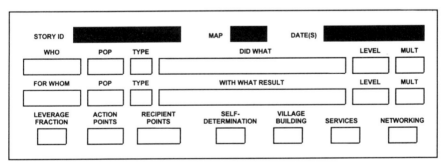

The first line of the map includes map identification information. The code for the story of which the map is a part (referred to as the STORY ID) is indicated. In the current example, the story has been named FRANCES. It might have been

---

[1] All the stories presented in this book are based on actual cases. However, they have each been altered somewhat to (a) serve as effective learning material in illustrating the points raised in the text and (b) protect the confidentiality of programs and clients.

called CLIENT 33, 97-033, or any other unique identifier selected by the program. The MAP CODE, which appears next, indicates the position of the map in the story sequence. The first map in the sequence is 1, the second 2, etc.[2] The DATE(S) field indicates the specific date when a service was provided or, for ongoing activity, the start and end dates of the activities covered in this particular map. For ongoing activities that will continue beyond the dates of the map, "++" is affixed to the end date (e.g., 11/97 to 2/98++).

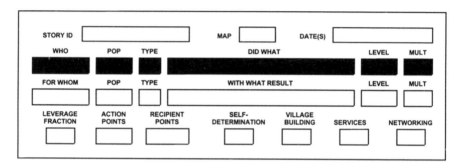

The second line of the map describes the actor or actors responsible for the activity being mapped and what they did. The WHO field names the actor or actors (referred to as the change agent). The POP field indicates how many change agents there were in this particular map. The TYPE field is a code used to describe the type of change agent (e.g., S stands for program staff; P for a single provider—not staff, and G for a group effort). In the DID WHAT field, the action taken is written (e.g., "delivered warm lunches to her home five times per week"). The LEVEL field is a code used to rate the relative impact potential of that action, as discussed in the next chapter. It begins with a prefix of either ACT (for action level) or MLS (for milestone level) followed by a rating from 1 to 7.

The MULT field is an integer that is multiplied by the LEVEL value and by the LEVERAGE FRACTION to produce the ACTION POINTS. When there is a single change agent, the MULT value is 1. When there are multiple change agents for the activity being mapped, the population multiplier conversion table is used to determine the value (see discussion in Chapter 6). However, this applies only when the change agent is a volunteer (with a TYPE code that begins with V, as with VS, VP, or VG). Otherwise, the MULT value is automatically 0 (i.e., no AC-TION POINTS are earned for a map when the change agents were paid to perform the activity).

---

[2] There are exceptions to this rule, such as labeling maps as MAP 0 or MAP 5b. These are explained in later chapters.

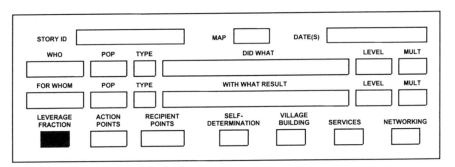

The third line of the map describes the recipients who are benefitting from the actions of the change agent. The FOR WHOM field names the recipient or recipients. The POP field indicates how many recipients there were in this particular map. The TYPE field is a code used to describe the type of recipient (e.g., C stands for the client featured in the story; F for a member of the client's family—when the entire family is not the client; and X for members of the program's target population other than the client or family members). In the WITH WHAT RESULT field, the immediate benefit of the action is written (e.g., "gained nourishment and social contact"). The LEVEL field is a code with the prefix LEV (for results level) followed by a rating from 1 to 5. That rating matches the one assigned to the change agent. Thus, ACT1 is matched with LEV1, ACT2 with LEV2, etc.

The MULT field is an integer that is multiplied by the LEVEL value and by the LEVERAGE FRACTION to produce the RECIPIENT POINTS. When there is a single recipient, the MULT value is 1. When there are multiple recipients for the activity being mapped, the population multiplier conversion table is used to determine the value (see discussion in Chapter 6).

The final row of the map begins with the LEVERAGE FRACTION. This number is used to possibly reduce the map score (a measure of the contribution of the program) when the change agent is not program staff nor has been in *direct* contact with staff in an earlier part of the story. For example, if a client shared new insights with a friend and then the friend used this knowledge to help others, the program would not get full credit for the map documenting the actions of the friend (and perhaps no credit). The leverage fraction would be either 0.5 or 0.0, depending on the type of program activity with the client that preceded the friend's actions.

| STORY ID | | MAP | | DATE(S) | | |
|---|---|---|---|---|---|---|

| WHO | POP | TYPE | DID WHAT | | LEVEL | MULT |
|---|---|---|---|---|---|---|
| | | | | | | |

| FOR WHOM | POP | TYPE | WITH WHAT RESULT | | LEVEL | MULT |
|---|---|---|---|---|---|---|
| | | | | | | |

| LEVERAGE FRACTION | ACTION POINTS | RECIPIENT POINTS | SELF-DETERMINATION | VILLAGE BUILDING | SERVICES | NETWORKING |
|---|---|---|---|---|---|---|
| | | | | | | |

The remaining fields in the map are used to display the points earned by the program for the contribution associated with the map. The values of earlier fields in the map are used to compute these points. The scoring algorithm is described in full in Chapter 6. The points can be calculated manually or be automatically computed using a simple spreadsheet or data base application.

Returning to Frances' story, the narrative suggested six direct or indirect program contributions to her health and life quality. These were:

Map 1.  Frances received warm lunches through the meals-on-wheels program operated by the senior center.

Map 2.  The volunteer who delivered the meals (John F.) encouraged her to visit the center after she got well.

Maps 3 and 4.  Frances benefitted from services and activities provided by the center's staff. (Two maps are used following a Results Mapping convention that no map should cover more than a three-month period.)

Map 5.  Frances attended the center on a regular basis. (This was considered a milestone in her life, as previously she had no contact with individuals her own age in Cincinnati.)

Map 6.  She has been volunteering in the kitchen helping to prepare the meals that the program delivers. (This marked an important role change for Frances from that of service recipient to a volunteer engaged in service provision—what we refer to as a "village builder" in Results Mapping.)

The formal mapping of these accomplishments would be as follows:

| STORY ID | FRANCES | | | MAP | 1 | DATE(S) | 3/97 TO 4/97 | |
|---|---|---|---|---|---|---|---|---|
| WHO | POP | TYPE | DID WHAT | | | | LEVEL | MULT |
| JOHN F. | 1 | VS | DELIVERED MEALS FIVE DAYS PER WEEK FOR 4 WEEKS | | | | ACT3 | 1 |
| FOR WHOM | POP | TYPE | WITH WHAT RESULT | | | | LEVEL | MULT |
| FRANCES | 1 | C | RECEIVED WARM, NUTRITIOUS FOOD AT HER HOME AND SOCIAL INTERACTION | | | | LEV3 | 1 |
| LEVERAGE FRACTION | ACTION POINTS | RECIPIENT POINTS | SELF-DETERMINATION | VILLAGE BUILDING | SERVICES | | NETWORKING | |
| 1.0 | 3 | 3 | 0 | 3 | 3 | | 0 | |

| STORY ID | FRANCES | | | MAP | 2 | DATE(S) | 4/97 | |
|---|---|---|---|---|---|---|---|---|
| WHO | POP | TYPE | DID WHAT | | | | LEVEL | MULT |
| JOHN F. | 1 | VS | ENCOURAGED HER TO VISIT THE CENTER | | | | ACT2 | 1 |
| FOR WHOM | POP | TYPE | WITH WHAT RESULT | | | | LEVEL | MULT |
| FRANCES | 1 | C | AGREED TO VISIT THE CENTER WHEN SHE GOT WELL | | | | LEV2 | 1 |
| LEVERAGE FRACTION | ACTION POINTS | RECIPIENT POINTS | SELF-DETERMINATION | VILLAGE BUILDING | SERVICES | | NETWORKING | |
| 1.0 | 2 | 2 | 0 | 2 | 2 | | 0 | |

| STORY ID | FRANCES | | | MAP | 3 | DATE(S) | 5/97 TO 7/97 | |
|---|---|---|---|---|---|---|---|---|
| WHO | POP | TYPE | DID WHAT | | | | LEVEL | MULT |
| PROGRAM STAFF | 2 | S | PROVIDED A RANGE OF ACTIVITIES AT THE CENTER | | | | ACT3 | 0 |
| FOR WHOM | POP | TYPE | WITH WHAT RESULT | | | | LEVEL | MULT |
| FRANCES | 1 | C | ENGAGED IN MULTIPLE ACTIVITIES ON REGULAR BASIS | | | | LEV3 | 1 |
| LEVERAGE FRACTION | ACTION POINTS | RECIPIENT POINTS | SELF-DETERMINATION | VILLAGE BUILDING | SERVICES | | NETWORKING | |
| 1.0 | 0 | 3 | 0 | 0 | 3 | | 0 | |

| STORY ID | FRANCES | | | MAP | 4 | DATE(S) | 8/97 TO 9/97++ | |
|---|---|---|---|---|---|---|---|---|
| WHO | POP | TYPE | DID WHAT | | | | LEVEL | MULT |
| PROGRAM STAFF | 2 | S | PROVIDED A RANGE OF ACTIVITIES AT THE CENTER | | | | ACT3 | 0 |
| FOR WHOM | POP | TYPE | WITH WHAT RESULT | | | | LEVEL | MULT |
| FRANCES | 1 | C | ENGAGED IN MULTIPLE ACTIVITIES ON REGULAR BASIS | | | | LEV3 | 1 |
| LEVERAGE FRACTION | ACTION POINTS | RECIPIENT POINTS | SELF-DETERMINATION | VILLAGE BUILDING | SERVICES | | NETWORKING | |
| 1.0 | 0 | 3 | 0 | 0 | 3 | | 0 | |

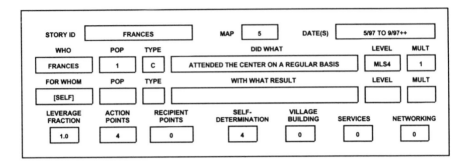

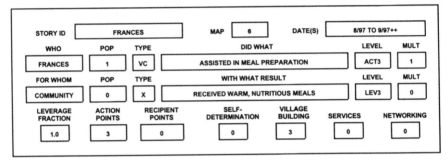

As earlier described, the core of each map of the story has the same grammar structure: [who] [did what] [for whom] [with what result]. In Map 5, where the actions taken were for self-benefit, the [with what result] section was left blank. Mapping conventions, as noted, dictate the time periods covered in the maps. Coding conventions determine the levels assigned to the action and recipient sections of each map. A scoring algorithm is used to translate these codes into action and recipient points; a classification system is used to convert these into self-determination, village building, or services/networking points. All this will become clear as we proceed. A concise summary of all the conventions can be found in Appendix B. Explanations for the codes and scoring of Frances' story can be found in Chapter 6.

No reference was made to outcomes in either the narrative or mapped accounts of Frances' story. Were these to be articulated, the outcomes associated with her ongoing story might include enhanced quality of life, continued independent living, and, should the need again arise, access to quality home assistance. As referenced several times, in Results Mapping, we focus on *contributions toward these outcomes* rather than on their attainment. Each map in the story was such a contribution, some more modest than others. The levels assigned to the maps (e.g., ACT3/LEV3 or MLS4) reflected the relative value of each contribution. Included were program contributions to the life of the client, as well as actions by the client herself that built on and were a follow-through to the program contributions.

With this brief background, let us return to the discussion of the five obstacles to the use of stories as evaluation data.

# TIME AND EFFORT

Once getting accustomed to the mapping procedure, it takes about ten minutes to map a story like the one just illustrated. What might take far more effort and time is finding the details of the story. In the illustration, this was relatively easy and quickly accomplished. Frances is a regular at the center and the fact that she attends regularly and has recently begun helping out in the kitchen is well known to the director and key staff at the senior center who provided the story. Furthermore, Frances' story did not involve a lot of twists and turns and the center was the only service provider. It gets far tougher to re-create a story where contact with the client has been lost and has to be re-established.

One might wonder how a program with one hundred or more active or recently served clients could possibly capture all the information needed for Results Mapping. Well the good news is that the program does not have to relate one story for each client. In fact, data from 12–15 stories are usually more than enough to gain a good sense of how the entire program operates to produce client growth—even where hundreds of clients have been served in recent years. But these cannot be just *any* dozen stories or a random sample of stories. They need to be the very best stories the program can provide (i.e., the stories that, when scored, receive the most points for program contributions and follow-through client actions).

It is quite common for programs to showcase their one or two most outstanding client success stories. It is much rarer for programs to array and analyze the dozen or so stories that feature their best work with clients. Yet these sets of top stories, when arrayed and analyzed, afford invaluable information regarding the practices of the programs. Further, should these programs be dedicated to continual improvement, there is perhaps no better data on which to base such improvement than that provided through study of their top stories.

Abraham Maslow reached a similar conclusion in his research on human potential. He noted that reports of the lives and work of geniuses were relatively common, while stories at the next tier of atypical individuals were rare. Maslow felt that a key to human advancement was linked to understanding better these individuals, whom he called high achievers or self-actualizers (Maslow, 1968). When asked why he did not expand his studies to more average persons, to get a more complete picture of human nature, Maslow's reported response was: "If you want to know what makes a runner fast, you do not waste time studying the techniques of slow runners."

In a similar spirit, Tom Peters and Robert Waterman rocked the business world with their lessons learned from studying the top-performing companies in their pursuits of excellence (Peters & Waterman, 1982). A similar strategy was applied by Osborne and Gaebler in their study of the public sector and the successful attempts there to re-invent government (Osborne & Gaebler, 1992).

For fix it/cure it programs, where all cases are supposed to be alike, the average case *is* a good place to start—since all cases ought to look like that case. However, for programs engaged in healing, transformation, and prevention, the average case offers little that the programs should want to emulate that is not also included in their better cases. But the reverse is not true. The average case lacks much that the better cases include. By drawing attention to a program's best work, it is our intention to prod that program to make the necessary adjustments so that the exceptional becomes the norm.

There is a second compelling reason why the best stories are enough for Results Mapping purposes. Because there has not been a focus by most programs on being exceptional, and because staff resources often have had to be spread thin among many clients, there simply are not that many exceptional stories that can be told. Once a program gets five or ten stories down in its story base, all the remaining stories tend to be rather "average." Put aside the few top stories, and the vast majority of programs engaged in healing and transformation take on the look of "fix it/cure it" programs. In short, they provide near identical services to clients and all their remaining stories sound pretty much the same.

The graph in Figure 2.1 illustrates this. The points earned by a representative program's best 15 stories are arrayed in descending order. The top two stories earned 50 and 42 points respectively. These are the stories that the program often uses to demonstrate its value. These are the anecdotes that make funders nervous. The next set of five stories earned points in the 30–20 range. Then there was another drop, with stories earning 14 points or less. The fifteenth best story the program could produce earned a scant 6 points. From service records, it appeared that there were 18 additional clients for whom stories might have been told (i.e., those for whom the program made at least some contribution during the previous two years). Further, were the program to map and score the "worst story" in the remaining group, it would have earned 2 points for a minor contribution to the client (e.g., the client was referred elsewhere and never heard from again).

The scores for the 18 stories below the top 15 can be estimated with reasonable confidence. They must range between 6 and 2 points. Using simple geometry, and assuming an even distribution of point values, the estimate of these points would be the sum of the two areas represented by the dotted triangle and rectangle in the figure. Thus, a "total score" for the program can be computed from its top stories, its worst story, and an estimate of how many stories there would be were all

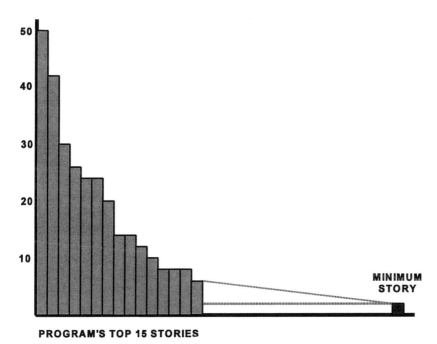

Figure 2.1. Points earned by a program's top stories. Note the dramatic drop in scores in the early stories and the leveling off of points that occurred by around the tenth best story. This is a common pattern.

stories in the client data base to be documented and scored. If a more informed estimation of the points for the remaining stories were desired, service records could be used to categorize the types of services received and likely client follow-through activities. Instead of a triangle, a step function would result, and the area under that function could easily be computed.

For programs engaged in institutional or systems-level change, this estimation procedure is typically unnecessary. Since Results Mapping is based on the last two years of performance (as discussed later), the total number of success stories that might be reported and mapped is generally low—likely fewer than 10. Hence, all program efforts should be mapped and included in the analysis.

So, in conclusion, programs are not required to devote excessive time and energy to storytelling and related research. A dozen or so complete stories are adequate—in most cases—for an end-of-the-year assessment of overall program performance. For the rare programs that have mastered the art of healing and transformation, and further have learned how to maximize local resources to serve lots of clients at exceptional levels, more stories (say, a total of 25–30) will be needed to derive a more complete picture of the best work of each such program.

But these are invariably the types of programs that keep in touch with their clients, know the stories, and—if need be—can get their clients to write their own stories and submit these for editing and analysis.

## STORYTELLING TECHNIQUE

The thorniest problem associated with Results Mapping is getting programs to report their work with clients clearly and completely. Once the details of a story are available, the mapping and associated scoring are easily accomplished by us or by others who have mastered the technique. When we first started asking programs to present their stories, we had little to offer them by way of examples or to serve as guides. Today, with several years of experience, reports, and story submissions from across the country to build upon, we can provide programs with clear examples of what a story needs to contain to be suitable for analysis. Many examples of this type appear in this book.

The rules governing mapping and scoring of stories are also helpful in guiding storytelling. The rules encourage a storyteller to explain simply and clearly how the program first got involved with the client, what actions it subsequently initiated to promote client health and growth, and how the client responded to these actions. When we return partially completed maps to programs with questions, and point out the rules that either have been violated or cannot be applied, they soon learn what it is we need and what is excessive or redundant reporting.

As an aid for those compiling data for stories, we have prepared a short questionnaire (refer to Appendix C). This instrument was designed for interactive use with a client (by telephone or in person) or as an organizer for a program staffer familiar with the story. It is not meant to serve as a stand-alone mail survey form because of its lack of user friendliness. When it is used with a client, we recommend that the client's story first be constructed in narrative form and then the questionnaire employed to capture the same information in a more structured manner.

## GETTING THE STORY STRAIGHT

Storytelling is a new endeavor for most programs. The information available in case notes, where these exist, can be very helpful in piecing together a story. For community development stories, there probably are no detailed case notes, and programs need to rely on memory, in-house monthly or quarterly reports, and the like as aids to story construction. Where networking with other service providers has occurred, these agencies should be contacted. They can help fill in details and add new information that the program may not have on record or otherwise know about.

Where clients can be contacted, programs are encouraged to do so. Programs need to stress to clients that: "They are being featured in a report on the *very best work of the program* in recent times. The program is proud of this work, as well as the growth that has taken place in the client, and wants to share this good news with others who may benefit from it." We know of no situations, so far, where clients did not want to have their stories told when presented in this light. In many cases, the process of having their stories told is self-validating and contributes further to the clients' transformations. They may ask to have identifying details removed or altered; and this can almost always be done to protect confidentiality and still produce stories that are close enough to the facts so that learning is not distorted and reported results remain valid.

One enterprising program in Milford, Connecticut, that prepares students to serve as "natural helpers" for peers with needs, used a group learning model to gather stories. Students were brought together in small groups and presented with examples of stories featuring other natural helpers. They were then asked to write narratives describing their own work and related impacts. They shared these with each other and answered questions from the group. This led to their adding key facts that they had left out of the initial narratives.

## CONSISTENCY ACROSS STORIES

The ability to present seemingly subjective and one-of-a-kind information in a standardized and systematic way that permits statistical analyses is what attracted me to Guttman's mapping sentence technology (referred to in the preface). Although our work has deviated considerably from that of Guttman and those who have continued to use and refine his approach, we have retained his core concept: using a standard mapping structure to report all key events that will subsequently be included in the analysis.

The narrative story represents an informal, somewhat unstructured account of the interactions between the program and the client (what might be classified as a "right brain dominant, left brain subordinate" reporting of the program–client interchange). The mapped story represents a formal, structured retelling of the account (i.e., a "left brain dominant, right brain subordinate" replay of that same interchange). It is as though a clever computer digests the narrative and reports it back emotion-free, logically, and linearly. We do not require consistency in the narrative accounts, provided there is sufficient detail to accomplish the mapping. One creative team from a Cincinnati senior center actually prepared some stories for us in poetic form. We have still not been handed a video, but I guess that is also a future possibility, particularly for a community development story.

We do, however, expect consistency in the mapped versions. Two individuals trained by us—or who have read and mastered the materials included in this book—when presented with a detailed narrative account, should map and score it in virtually the same way. There is some room for interpretation during mapping, but very little. A particular map, for example, might be assigned a raw score of 2 by one mapper and a score of 3 by the second; but this will have little bearing on the analysis that follows or on the conclusions drawn—unless there are many maps of this type in the program's story set. Where significant mapping differences have arisen in the past, we have invariably modified a mapping rule or convention to eliminate these differences and regain consistency across mappers.

# AGGREGATING THE INFORMATION

The coding and related scoring system associated with Results Mapping are what set it apart from other forms of program evaluation of which we are aware (but I am again reminded of King Solomon's pronouncement that "there is nothing truly new under the sun" and will not be surprised if comparable work exists). Each program action that directly or indirectly encourages growth of the client featured in a story receives a code and score. Linked actions by other service providers or family/community members that benefit that client are also coded and scored, as is each action taken by the client for self-help or to benefit some other person(s) with similar needs. As scores for a story accumulate, these are subtotaled as service, networking, village building, and self-determination points.

Among these codes, a special set are called "milestones." These are akin to short-term and intermediate-range outcomes associated with more traditional evaluation approaches. In the story illustrated earlier, Frances reached a short-term outcome (coded as MLS4) when she began participating in activities at the senior center on a regular basis. This was significant in her life, since she was new to the city and had few acquaintances in her own age range. The new habit of going to the center certainly added to her quality of life. If the program continues to map Frances's story, at some point soon she will be credited with reaching MLS6, a sustained, intermediate-range outcome.

The combination of codes, milestones reached, and points—within and across stories—provides a comprehensive picture of the best work of a program. A very effective total quality improvement system emerges when a program begins to track these data from one evaluation period to the next, while taking steps to increase the levels of activity, numbers of client milestones reached, and point productivity in its top stories.

With due caution, agencies that operate multiple programs—each aimed at different target populations pursuing varied and different outcomes—can contrast the action levels, client milestones, and point productivity associated with each program and draw conclusions regarding their relative effectiveness as agents of healing and transformation. Similarly, funders providing resources to varied programs can begin to see where they are getting most impact—via program contributions toward short-term and longer-term client outcomes—for their dollars. Care must be taken to relate findings of program differences to factors such as client readiness, contextual variables (e.g., culture and political climate), program experience, adequacy of resources, and existence of best practices and well-researched strategies that can be adapted locally. Still, it is important to begin to make these comparisons so that reasonable pressure can be placed on programs to make the most of the resources with which they have been entrusted.

# QUIZ 2

2.1. Why does Results Mapping focus on a program's *best* stories? Wouldn't we get more reliable information regarding the overall program by random sampling? Also, shouldn't a program's *worse* stories be studied to discover what the program is doing wrong and needs to correct?

2.2. Why do total quality management principles (e.g., working for zero defects, visible measures of performance, and shared responsibility for quality output) work better when applied to factory production systems than to social service or prevention programs?

2.3. Is it possible to be "objective" when the unit of analysis is a story? Are numbers inherently more objective than stories?

# 3

# The Results Ladder

*The stage model is one of the most widely used tools in Western psychology. It has been fruitfully applied to psychosexual, cognitive, ego, moral, affective, object-relational, and linguistic lines of development—in short, to virtually the entire gamut of development studied by conventional psychology and psychiatry (Wilber, Engler, & Brown, 1986, p. 4).*

There are fundamental laws and patterns of behavior governing our universe. In the realm of physical interactions, for example, there is the law of attraction between two bodies:

$$A_{12} = M_1 \times M_2/D_{12}^2$$

where the extent of attraction ($A_{12}$) is directly related to the relative mass ($M_1$ and $M_2$) of the two objects and inversely related to the square of the distance ($D_{12}$) separating the two.

Economists make extensive use of the laws of diminishing returns on investment and the interplay—in a free economy—of supply and demand. Geographers apply the principles of central place theory to explain how cities, towns, and villages are arranged in space.

Various investigators of the creative process in science or the arts have observed four stages in a vast majority of creative breakthroughs—across cultures and disciplines (Harmon & Rheingold, 1984):

**Stage 1 [Preparation]:** Hours, days, and sometimes years of experimentation and investigatory effort occur in which the individual (or team) feels close to a breakthrough but cannot break through.

Stage 2 [Incubation]: The individual takes time away from the challenge to think about other things, go on vacation, or simply catch a few hours of needed sleep.

Stage 3 [Illumination]: A sudden and clear vision of the solution enlightens the individual, typically made possible by an amazingly simple shift of perspective.

Stage 4 [Verification]: The individual determines that the Aha! moment was in fact a breakthrough by applying it successfully to the task at hand.

In the realm of psychology, Abraham Maslow outlined a hierarchy of needs through which all individuals progress on their way to optimum psychological health (Figure 3.1) (Maslow, 1968). At level 1, basic needs for food, shelter, and safety are addressed. At level 2, individuals need and seek love and a sense of belonging. At level 3, they wish to be acknowledged and appreciated for their contributions to family, group, or society. At level 4, they strive for "self-actualization" as individuals at peace within themselves and appreciative of what life has offered and continues to offer to them. At level 5, they reach beyond the psychological limits of self to earn a sense of oneness and wholeness within the totality of human existence and experience.

There appears also to be a hierarchy of levels that individuals, groups, or communities invariably pass through on their path toward transformation and healing. This is analogous to but different from the stages and hierarchy just described. We refer to it as the *Results Ladder*. This Ladder (Figure 3.2) is the spine around which Results Mapping has been constructed.

Allow me to use a fictional example to introduce the Results Ladder:

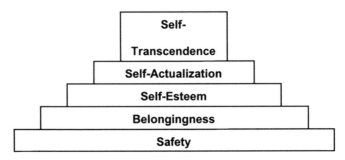

Figure 3.1. Maslow's hierarchy of needs. The individual can pursue higher-order needs for self-actualization and self-transcendency only after the basic needs, at the lower levels, have been satisfied.

Barney was a couch potato. Each evening, he arrived home from work, ate dinner, and plopped down on the sofa to watch hours of television. In the world around him—on television, in the magazine articles he read, and in the form of the joggers and striders he regularly saw on the streets of his town—were continual messages warning of the dangers of a sedentary life style. Through these many indirect, public messages, Barney knew he ought to exercise. But he chose not to do so. He was operationally at Level 1 of the Results Ladder.

About a year ago, Barney spotted a former high school classmate, Albert, whom he had not seen in years. And Albert looked simply marvelous, years younger than his age. Barney had to ask, "How come you look so good, Albert? Are you coloring your hair?" Albert laughed. "Oh, no. Believe it or not, a year ago I looked as bad as you do. Then I started working out. It's made all the difference in the world." As he jogged off, Albert turned and shouted, "You ought to try

Figure 3.2. The Results Ladder. Included are seven levels, three of which are designated as milestones because they represent sustained behavior adjustments toward longer-term outcomes.

| |
|---|
| **MILESTONE 7**<br>Attained mastery level<br>in personal growth area<br>(lifetime achievement) |
| **MILESTONE 6**<br>Made and sustained<br>positive adjustment<br>(at least six months) |
| **LEVEL 5**<br>Received on-going support<br>[while assuming increased<br>personal responsibility] |
| **MILESTONE 4**<br>Made short-term,<br>positive adjustment<br>(at least one month) |
| **LEVEL 3**<br>Received routine,<br>short-term service |
| **LEVEL 2**<br>Received personalized advice<br>via direct contact |
| **LEVEL 1**<br>Received general information<br>via indirect means |

it. There's a fitness center in town where I work out that is offering a free trial membership. Drop by."

Barney was at Level 2. He had still taken no action, but had received personalized advice and been directed to a course of possible action.

Barney figured that he didn't have much to lose by taking advantage of the free offer. He drove to the fitness center, wandered in, and looked around. He was intimidated. Too many muscles and too much sweat for his sensitivities. He turned to leave.

"Hi! I'm Tony, can I help you?" Barney turned toward the voice, and eyed a young, muscular guy with a smile. They conversed a few minutes, and Barney received assurances that it was in fact a free offer without strings, that there were a series of beginning classes and training available throughout the week, and that he would not be the only out-of-shape person taking part in these.

Barney made three trips to the fitness center during the next week and discovered, to his surprise, that he liked the exercises and activities and could perform better than he thought he could. Tony and the other staff proved to be very helpful and encouraging. Barney was now at Level 3: he had received a short-term, routine service pointing him in the direction of better health.

The next step was critical. Barney had to make a decision about whether to move forward or not. He decided to sign up for three months at the center and rearranged his schedule so that he could get to the center at least four times each week. This demanded that he make some adjustments in his life style, including getting off the sofa and exercising for a few hours each week. He was far from being a fitness buff, but at least he had taken the plunge. During that three-month period, Barney attended the center on a regular basis. He found classes he enjoyed and a particular trainer whom he sought out regularly for advice and assistance. He also began reading books on nutrition and modified his diet. He had reached Milestone 4.

By the time the three-month membership had expired, Barney was well on his way to maintaining a life based on fitness and health. He paid in advance for a year's membership and became a regular at the center. He worked out at the center an average of four days each week throughout the next year. He made friends with a small group at the center who liked to go hiking on weekends and soon was participating with them in these outings. Barney was now at Level 5.

Barney set a personal goal to run a mile in under six minutes. This goal was achieved eight months later. A party was held to celebrate this new milestone (Milestone 6).

As of this writing, Barney remains committed to his new life-style. He has begun cycling and has plans to compete in the Senior Olympics in some event by the year 2003. He dreams of winning a gold medal in his age class. Should he advance to this level of fitness and athletic prowess, whether he wins the medal or not, Barney will have reached Milestone 7.

To summarize Barney's transformation (from bottom to top):

Milestone 7. Reaps and demonstrates the full benefits of new lifestyle
Milestone 6. Fully adjusted to new lifestyle/status
Level 5. Received advanced services/coaching/sustained support
Milestone 4. Demonstrated commitment to change
Level 3. Received short-term, routine service
Level 2. Obtained personal advice and an option
Level 1. Exposed to general information and warnings

As discussed briefly in the Preface, when we first introduced Results Mapping in 1995, a major, early step in the implementation process was the development of a unique set of hierarchies for each new application. For example, to evaluate five family resource centers in Cincinnati, we constructed prevention, emergency services, direct services, and institution-building hierarchies. Over the next two years, as many as two dozen different sets of results hierarchies were developed through interactions with funders, program staff, client representatives, and content experts. In May 1997, after I had just spent a day developing yet another customized set of hierarchies, it suddenly dawned on me that there was, in fact, a single underlying hierarchy. The two dozen unique sets of hierarchies were actually variations of the same Ladder. I plotted out The Results Ladder and, as I suspected, it fit neatly over each one of these variations. Where there were differences, these were minor and could easily be adjusted to match the hierarchy presented here.

Although the Results Ladder is an original template for describing stages of progress toward healing and transformation, not surprisingly it somewhat resembles other hierarchies that have been developed to capture change and growth processes. To illustrate:

**Maslow's hierarchy of needs.** The bottom rung of Maslow's hierarchy, where basic needs are recognized and met, is similar to the lower three levels of the Results Ladder. A sense of belonging, his second level, fits Milestone 4; self-esteem, if sustained and translated to practice, roughly corresponds to Level 5; self-actualization mirrors Milestone 6; and self-transcendence would correspond with Milestone 7. Maslow noted that most persons seem content to remain at the middle levels and do not strive toward self-actualization and self-transcendence. In our own work, we have observed that most program activities and services operate at or below Level 3, supporting, at best, short-term, positive life adjustments by clients (our Milestone 4). In the absence of services and results at Level 5, most program clients do not progress to Milestones 6 and 7, mirroring a similar glass ceiling effect to that noted by Maslow.

**The precaution adoption model.** The precaution adoption model in public health is used to explore how individuals adjust to perceived hazards (Weinstein & Sandman, 1992). Under that model, the individual first becomes aware from the media that there is a hazard (our Level 1). He initially concludes that it is a threat to others, but not to self (Level 2). He realizes, through more study, that he too is at risk (Level 3). He makes a short-term adjustment to reduce personal risk (Milestone 4). He sustains these changes over time (Milestone 6) by making permanent changes in his life style or living conditions (Level 5).

**Health and healing.** In his currently popular writings on health and healing, Andrew Weil contends that healing comes from inside, not outside. He states, "Medicines and medicine men can sometimes catalyze a healing response or remove obstructions to it, but they never give you what you do not already have." Weil posits that many successful medical interventions (our Level 3) are actually *active placebos* that increase both the doctor's and client's beliefs in the possibility of healing (Weil, 1983; 1995). The strength of the client's belief (Milestone 4) then somehow activates the client's innate healing abilities (Level 5), increasing the odds of recovery of fuller health (Milestone 6).

When introducing Results Mapping to a new program, we first present the Results Ladder and then identify results the program achieves with its clients that fall under each of the levels and milestones of the Ladder. On the chart on the next pages (Table 3.1) are examples from a variety of programs where the approach has been implemented. These are discussed, in turn, below.

The first example, physical fitness, was played out in Barney's story, which I used above to introduce the Results Ladder. Note that at Level 2 a different type of activity is used as an illustration (i.e., attended a health fair and talked to a nurse). In general, there can be a variety of actions and consequences that fit each rung of the Ladder. With practice, it becomes relatively easy to select the level or milestone that applies to each situation being mapped. Aids to making these selections are provided later in this chapter.

The second example, substance abuse prevention, examines the progress of a youngster (or group of youth) in accepting responsibility for personal decisions and moving toward responsible behavior regarding use of drugs (as broadly defined to include alcohol, tobacco, marijuana, cocaine, etc.) Note the distance (three or more levels) separating information, motivation, and short-term training from Milestone 6—a long-term goal for a substance abuse prevention program.

**Table 3.1.** Applications of the Results Ladder to Diverse Social and Health Transformations[a]

| Level | Physical fitness | Substance abuse prevention | Accessing quality health care | Coalition functioning | Independent living |
|---|---|---|---|---|---|
| MLS7 | Earned a medal in the Senior Olympics for cycling or running | Established and led a motivational group that promoted drug-free lifestyles | Dramatically improved health, wellness, or quality-of-life status (at least two years) | A major policy change was achieved in an issue area of vital importance to the coalition | Able to maintain an apartment and live fully within the community through age 95+ |
| MLS6 | Attained and maintained personal health and fitness goals (at least six months) | Remained drug-free throughout high school | Incrementally improved health, wellness, or quality-of-life status (at least six months) | Coalition obtained key resources and fully implemented long-range strategy | Secured assistance that allowed long-term residence in a preferred living environment |
| LEV5 | Received ongoing coaching or training with regard to personal health and fitness (at least three months) | Participated on regular basis in supervised drug-free group activity (e.g., sports club) | Working with doctor, found diet and stress relief that activated the healing process | [Coalition task force] received ongoing technical assistance from a national expert in a key issue area | Served as secretary-treasurer for condo complex |
| MLS4 | Began regular exercise routine / more healthy diet (maintained for more than one month) | Signed contract agreeing not to experiment with drugs and kept to its terms for more than one month | Began managing with assistance own health care needs / gained faith in healing prospects | [Coalition task force] completed development of action plan for meeting short-term goals of coalition | Began attending the local senior center on a regular basis and participating in its meals program |

(continued)

**Table 3.1.** (*Continued*)

| Level | Physical fitness | Substance abuse prevention | Accessing quality health care | Coalition functioning | Independent living |
|---|---|---|---|---|---|
| LEV3 | Received instruction in some health or fitness activity | Received training in refusal skills (to overcome peer pressures) | Screened for potential problem or accessed and received needed services | [Coalition members] received training in recruitment of diverse groups (e.g., youth and seniors) | Provided with a needed, ongoing service (e.g., transportation) to permit regular access to places outside the home |
| LEV2 | Attended a health fair and talked with a nurse about the value of folic acid and vitamin E | Listened to motivational speaker in small classroom setting | Received specific knowledge about how to access a service | [Local agency director] received personal call with request to contribute resources to coalition | Discussed availability of adult day services, home care, meals on wheels, or daily wellness checks |
| LEV1 | Received information pertaining to wellness or fitness [passive learning] | Exposed to warning messages on television about dangers of drug use | Received directory of health resources that are available in the community | [Community members] learned about activities of the coalition through media | Received pamphlets or other information regarding resources available to promote or enhance independence |

[a]Note that these are examples and not the only services or activities that could fit into the various cells of the table.

This demonstrates graphically what research in this area has concluded: information, motivation, and brief training alone are unlikely to produce significant, lasting effects on drug-related decisions and actions of youth exposed to them (Stewart & Klitzner, 1992). It further shows the value of program activities that bring clients to Level 5 (e.g., their engagement in mentoring programs and long-term healthy alternatives) and, hence, within reach of the goal.

The third example, accessing quality health care, is similar to the first example. The individuals progressing along the Results Ladder are seeking an end to their illness or suffering and a restoration of quality of health. At the lower levels, they obtain information, gain advice and/or are directed to healing resources, and receive routine services. Beginning with Milestone 4, they begin to take personal responsibility for their healing and, at Level 5, receive the personalized attention that builds hope, confidence, and strength.

The fourth example, coalition functioning, indicates levels reached in attracting new members and preparing them with needed skills for effective participation in the coalition. At the two advanced levels (Milestone 6 and Milestone 7), a member of the coalition—or more likely the entire team—achieved success in advancing the mission of the coalition by obtaining key resources and catalyzing new public policy. In interpreting the Results Ladder for this example, progress of the "coalition" needs to be viewed flexibly to cover advances of some of its members, task forces, or perhaps issues promoted by the coalition.

In the final example—independent living—growth is plotted in the capacities of older adults to remain in the community despite challenges associated with aging. Note that this is just one pathway to Milestone 7. Older adults need not participate in a senior center to reach Milestone 4, for example. Nor do they need to be officers in their condo complex to operate at Level 5.

An expanded version of the Results Ladder is presented in Figure 3.3.

| MLS7 | | |
|------|---|---|
| MLS6 | | |
| ACT5 | ➤ | LEV5 |
| MLS4 | | |
| ACT3 | ➤ | LEV3 |
| ACT2 | ➤ | LEV2 |
| ACT1 | ➤ | LEV1 |

Figure 3.3. The expanded Results Ladder. Here both the actions of change agents and the parallel progress of clients can be tracked.

As can be seen, the expanded Ladder includes the same seven levels and milestones. However, it emphasizes the role of an additional actor, the *change agent*, in assisting the client (or other recipients included in the client's story) to reach Levels 1, 2, 3, and 5. The use of a dual system of coding (ACTn and LEVn/MLSn) is key to Results Mapping, since the program being evaluated plays this role of change agent for its clients. These clients start out as recipients but can evolve to change agents, in their own right, for self and others.

Allow me to discuss the four action levels, after which I will return to the three milestones:

At Level 1, the change agent produces and distributes public information (ACT1) that reaches the client indirectly as one member of the target audience (LEV1).

**Example:** The federal government spent $195 million on anti-drug advertising spots during the most watched television hours. The target was youth. This was an ACT1 activity that yielded a LEV1 result for the youth who were exposed to these spots.

At Level 2, the change agent motivates, prods, offers advice, and makes referrals (ACT2) to which the client may or may not respond (LEV2).

**Example:** A famous professional basketball player returned to his former high school to address the student body. He encouraged the students to study hard and stay away from drugs and alcohol. Following his presentation, he responded to questions posed by the students and teachers. The speaker was functioning at ACT2 and having a LEV2 impact on his audience.

**Example:** The program referred one of its clients, who is a problem drinker, to a support group in town. The referral was an ACT2, the immediate effect of the referral on the client was at LEV2.

**Example:** A client, on her own, got on the Internet to seek tips for giving up smoking. She received over 80 responses. This was an action for self-benefit at ACT2, with no separate recipient (and hence no matching LEV2 code).

At Level 3, the change agent delivers routine services or helps build client skills (ACT3) that produce short-term client status changes (LEV3).

**Example:** Dr. Franklin, to whom the client had been referred by the parish nurse, examined her and confirmed that her blood pressure was dangerously low as the nurse had suspected. He prescribed a change in medication. The doctor's service was at ACT3, the benefit to the client was at LEV3.

Example: The Salvation Army provided warm meals, twice daily, to homeless persons in town. This was an ACT3 service benefitting those receiving the meals at LEV3.

Example: A group of 12 students were picked by the program to attend a leadership training retreat. During a three-day period, they interacted with 200 other youth and gained a set of new skills for mobilizing their peers back home. The coordinators of the retreat were functioning at ACT3, while the 12 youth (as well as the 200 others who perhaps were being mapped in some other programs' stories) were benefitting at LEV3.

Example: A new coalition to tackle local environmental health issues met weekly for two months to establish priorities and plan promotional activities. This was an ACT3 effort for future community benefit. Since there were no recipients as yet, there was no matching LEV3 assigned.

At Level 5, the change agent plays the role of coach or advisor to the client (ACT5) to support the latter's activities and sustained growth (LEV5). The intention of the change agent is to shift the locus of control for sustained growth to the client (i.e., to empower the client to guide his or her own transformation process).

Example: A 4-H club leader coordinated weekly group activities over a two-year period. During that period, eight club members were encouraged to take on projects for which they won blue ribbons. The leader functioned at ACT5 to benefit the club members at LEV5 (who reached MLS6).

Example: A mother provided intensive, around-the-clock care for her ailing son during a prolonged illness that lasted eight months. As her son's condition improved, he was able to take on increased responsibility for his own care and return to full health. She was acting at ACT5 to benefit her son at LEV5.

Example: A corporate executive on loan to United Way for one year oversaw the launching and implementation of a major new funding initiative. As the year went by, he trained and turned over more responsibilities to other community volunteers. He was acting at ACT5. The other volunteers were benefitting at LEV5.

Example: A senior citizen recovering from heart surgery began speed walking as part of his recovery regimen. During the next two years, he built up his speed and endurance to the point where he was competing well in local races. He was acting at ACT5 for self-benefit (and reached MLS6). There would be no LEV5 associated with his efforts (i.e., the change agent *is* the recipient).

Example: A local school district, with the guidance of the program, converted from a traditional to an open systems environment. Within three years, students were routinely engaged in peer learning, work-study programs, and varied community service projects. A rich array of learning experiences were being provided by community-based business persons, artists, and craftspeople. The school district was engaged in an ACT5 transformation for community benefit that led to its reaching MLS6. (Note: This would be a complicated story to map. In addition to several maps showing interactions among the school population—as change agents and recipients—there would be a global map indicating that the school district itself had advanced to ACT5 activity—with no recipient—and another map showing it attaining MLS6.)

The easiest way to distinguish between ACT1→LEV1 and ACT2→LEV2 is through the directness of the relationship between the change agent and the client. At Level 1, the change agent is targeting efforts at the general public and not at any specific client. At Level 2, the change agent is focused directly on a specific client's progress or health. Note the client can be an individual or a group.

The primary distinction between ACT2→LEV2 and ACT3→LEV3 is in the role the change agent plays for the client. At Level 2, that role is one of prodder and referral source. At Level 3, it is to actually mend, educate, train, or otherwise cause short-term improvements in the client's status. Again, the client can be an individual or a group.

The main difference between ACT3→LEV3 and ACT5→LEV5 is in the nature of the relationship between the client and the change agent. At Level 3, the change agent leads and the client follows. It is a teacher–student, parent–child, or doctor–patient relationship. At Level 5, the relationship transforms to adult-adult (to employ the terminology of Eric Berne's transactional analysis; Berne, 1964) or from an I–it to an I–Thou relationship (to use Martin Buber's paradigm; Buber, 1992) and the role of the change agent is gradually reduced to allow the client to move forward to MLS6. If the client is an institution or a system, Level 3 activity tends to be preparatory work (e.g., a series of planning meetings), whereas Level 5 activity relates to full program implementation (e.g., carrying out the plan).

At Milestones 4, 6, and 7, there are no external change agents (and hence no ACT codes). The client—always an individual or single entity (e.g., a school system)—is acting as a self-change agent. Let me review each of the three:

At MLS4, the client (or a close relation to the client whose behavior is critical to the growth or health of the client) has shifted from passive to active mode. The individual has received enough information, prodding, advice, and routine services from others to recognize the need for personal change and has taken first steps in this direction. At least one month of changed behavior is required, by convention, to credit the individual with this milestone.

Example: An individual followed his doctor's suggestions and began eating a restricted, fat-reduced diet.

Example: A problem drinker started attending meetings of Alcoholics Anonymous on a regular basis.

Example: A task force completed the planning phase and began implementing its action alternatives.

Example: Students signed a contract declaring that they would not drink alcoholic beverages and reported, two months later, that they had not touched a drink although they had been to parties where other students were drinking and encouraging them to do likewise.

At MLS6, the client has become more self-sufficient and can point to marked increases in health, positive behavior, or fullness of being. By convention, the new behavior will have been sustained for more than six months and been preceded by at least one earlier map in the story at results level 5 with a program staffer or staff volunteer serving as the change agent. In addition, the client will have some achievement to point to as evidence of a fundamental change in behavior or status.

Example: A former welfare recipient maintained a job for eight months *and* was recommended by her supervisor for a major promotion.

Example: A 16-year-old with a history of discipline and truancy problems turned over a new leaf, completed his junior year without incidents or unexcused absences, *and* made the school B honor roll for the first time.

Example: A state prevention agency re-invented itself as a consumer-centered, asset-building support system for local programs and organizations. *And* it was able to demonstrate, using Results Mapping, that it had doubled its contributions toward intermediate-level outcomes in the State in one year with the same operating budget.

At MLS7, the client is recognized by self and others as an advanced practitioner in areas associated with the outcome(s) being targeted by the program. Some truly outstanding achievement is needed as demonstration that this milestone has been reached.

Example: A former bank robber and drug dealer, having served prison time and returned to college to complete his education, earned a Ph.D. in criminology and wrote an award-winning book on his life and lessons learned.

Example: A group of former welfare moms established an "e-business," with support from IBM and the program, and achieved $16 million dollars in sales in their second full year of operation.

Example: An individual who had been in institutional care most of his adult life for mental illness became a deacon of his church, held down a full-time job, and met and married a woman whom he loves dearly.

Example: A hospital-based clinic for the practice of integrative medicine transformed into a "clinic without walls" by building, in collaboration with more than one hundred partners, a county-wide network of support agencies and traditional and non-traditional practitioners.

The main difference between MLS4 and MLS6 is the intensity of commitment of the client and the extent to which changes have been integrated into the client's life. This is typically measured by the length of time that the client has sustained these changes. At MLS4, the client is testing the waters (at least one month) with no long-term commitment. At MLS6, the client has a multi-month (at least six months) history of personal engagement in the healing or transformation process and can point to sustained gains in health, wellness, or life quality.

The main difference between MLS6 and MLS7 is that the latter represents a total integration of the changes the client has been seeking and inducing. The work is complete, no relapse is anticipated or likely. If further change does occur, it will be along an entirely new growth path. The caterpillar has become a butterfly.

These three milestones are the *outcome levels* that funders and programs are most interested in seeing clients reach. MLS4 can be viewed as a short-term or intermediate outcome, MLS6 as a longer-term outcome, and MLS7 as an ultimate or ideal outcome. The earlier levels (particularly gains at LEV3) can be viewed as initial outcomes that often are necessary precursors to higher-level development.

Different funders employ slightly different terminology to define varied levels of outcome. United Way of America, for example, suggests use of initial, intermediate, and longer-term outcomes (Table 3.2). San Francisco Bay Area United Way agencies have been trained to use intermediate and long-term outcomes and distinguish for these two time-based results between individual, community, and system-change outcomes. The integration of these milestones with ACTs and LEVs allows a full picture to emerge of the actions and responses needed to bring clients toward and to these desired outcome levels.

**Table 3.2.** Correspondence between Milestones and United Way Outcomes

| Results Ladder | United Way of America outcomes |
| --- | --- |
| LEV3 | Initial outcomes |
| MLS4 | Intermediate outcomes |
| MLS6 | Longer-term outcomes |
| MLS7 | Ultimate outcomes |

# QUIZ 3

3.1. Johnny viewed a public service announcement on television that warned against the use of chewing tobacco. *What level did this represent for him?*

3.2. The team put up anti-drug posters around the school. *What was this action level?*

3.3. Dave, a recovering alcoholic, established a support group for co-workers from his office that meets weekly. Dave reported having reached his first anniversary without a drink. *What was the personal milestone level reached by Dave? When can support group members begin receiving milestones for their accomplishments? At what milestone level?*

3.4. Dr. Smith suggested that Sally call the child care center to seek placement for her child. *At what action level was Dr. Smith operating? What was the benefit level for Sally?*

3.5. Marie, who had not been following her doctor's advice regarding her diet, almost died. Following an emergency intervention, she began monitoring her diet closely and has not had a recurring medical problem in nine months. *What levels has she been operating at during these nine months and what personal milestones has she reached?*

3.6. Jennie is a fantastic trainer. She conducted a three-hour workshop for 15 trainees. Larry, a boring trainer, conducted the same three-hour workshop for 15 different trainees. *At what action level was Jennie operating? At what action level was Larry operating?*

3.7. Frank agreed to serve as a mentor for young Arnie. For a year, he met with Arnie three times a week to help with reading and homework and to take Arnie on outings to museums and sporting events. Arnie often initiates calls to Frank for advice and is now talking about becoming a mentor for a younger child. *What level of relationship developed between Frank and Arnie by the end of the year? Is there any indication of a milestone for Arnie and, if so, at what level?*

3.8. Maurice suffers from Alzheimer's disease. He has attended an adult day center daily for the past eight months, where he spends his day being a passive recipient of services. Thanks to the center, his daughter, who is Maurice's primary care giver, has been able to keep her job and get some respite. *What is the highest milestone Maurice can reach? What milestone has his daughter reached?*

3.9. On the July 4th weekend, the local police were out in force checking for intoxicated drivers. *At what level were they operating? Who were their "clients"?*

# Terminology and Key Mapping Concepts

Results Mapping is used to map, score, analyze, and provide feedback to improve the best work that a program does with its clients, be these individuals, families, teams, groups, communities, organizations, or systems. Each story features some of that best work. It is not the client's life story that is being presented. Nor is it only the interface of the program with the client. Rather, it is a story that *begins* with the first interaction between the program and the client and *extends* to further program-client interactions, to program interactions with the client's support system, to client interchanges with others called on by the program to assist the client, *and* to personal client achievements in support of self or to benefit others.

Excluded from the story are services provided to the client by other agencies that are not linked to earlier program actions to benefit the client. Also excluded are client activities and achievements that are not linked to the program's objectives *or* are well beyond the contributions of the program to these achievements (see discussion of leveraging in Chapter 6).

## CL-I-ENT NOT CLIENT

Rather than produce outcomes, the programs whose work is best suited for study through Results Mapping are helping their clients grow out of the circumstances that diminish their lives and into new life contexts. To keep reminding us of this as we proceed, I will begin using the term cl-I-ent in the materials that follow. The capital "I" emphasizes that the program is working with subjects, not objects, to foster self-determination, growth, health, and emergence of creative potential. This convention will be followed for all types of cl-I-ents, be they indiv-

I-duals, fam-I-lies, un-I-ts, ne-I-ghborhoods, commun-I-ties, organ-I-zations, or inst-I-tutions.

## TYPES OF MAPS

A story relates how the program being evaluated has contributed to near-term and longer-term cl-I-ent successes both directly and through leveraging the resources of others (including those of the cl-I-ent). That story is told in narrative form (by a program representative, the cl-I-ent, or both) and then mapped and scored using a formalized method. Each element of the mapped story is referred to as a mapping sentence or simply as a *map*.

There are two types of maps used to document a story. The more common type is a *transactional map*. A transactional map has this form:

Here there is both a change agent and a recipient.[1] The *change agent* may be a staff member of the program, but could also be staff from another program, a volunteer, a member of the cl-I-ent's family, the cl-I-ent (in support of others), or anyone else taking actions to benefit a recipient. The *recipient* may be the cl-I-ent, a family member, or another community member benefitting from the actions of the change agent; or a future change agent that is being mobilized to action.

Example: Jane, a staffer, provided 6 hours of training for 15 youth. [Jane is the change agent and the 15 youth are the recipients.]
Example: The 15 youth shared lessons from the training with 20 peers. [The 15 youth—recipients in an earlier map—are now the change agents and their 20 peers are the recipients of this map.]

---

[1] For general discussion throughout the remainder of the book, singular tense will be used unless those being discussed are clearly plural in number. Thus, for example, I will talk about the change agent rather than change agent(s) and a recipient rather than recipient(s).

Example: Tom, a staffer, referred the cl-I-ent to the local housing authority. [Tom is the change agent and the housing authority is the recipient of this map.] Note that we refer to this kind of transaction as a *handoff* that earns the program "networking points," as discussed below.

The second type of map is a *self-referential map*. A self-referential map has this form:

Here there is a change agent but no recipient. In effect, the change agent is the recipient, taking action for self-benefit. This type of map is also used when the change agent is taking action that ultimately is meant to benefit another, but when that benefit will only accrue after subsequent action is taken.

Example: Harry joined the local YMCA and is swimming a mile each morning in its lap pool. [Harry was the change agent, but there was no recipient.]

Example: The task force spent six months developing an action plan. [The task force was the change agent, but there was no recipient. Future maps, documenting how the plan is implemented, would likely be transactional.]

# MAP SEQUENCE

Maps are presented in roughly chronological order to capture all significant contributions of the program to current and future cl-I-ent successes. Again, these include contributions where program staff are the change agent but also contributions made through the efforts of others that can be linked back to earlier, related program efforts. For complex stories involving many maps and possibly several different outcomes, it is sometimes easier and clearer to group maps dealing with a particular outcome or associated service. This may lead to the entire set of maps of the story not being presented in strict chronological order.

# MAP CODES

For transactional maps, each change agent action is coded (with an ACTn) as is each recipient response (with a LEVn). For self-referential maps, where there is no recipient, only the change agent action is coded (as an MLSn or ACTn). For transactional maps, the results level (n) is the same for both the ACTn and the LEVn codes. Thus, for example, if the action taken is coded as ACT1, then the gain to the recipient must be LEV1. The values of n range from 1 through 7.

There are seven *results levels* (as introduced in the previous chapter). They are used to categorize the type of action taken by the change agent and the matching benefit to the recipient. Three of these levels only appear on self-referential maps (and are distinguished from the others by changing the ACTn code to a MLSn code—for personal "milestone"). The remaining four levels may appear on both transactional and self-referential maps, although they are far more common in transactional maps. For self-referential maps, the information or services at ACT2, ACT3, and ACT5 are self-provided. Thus, for example, ACT3 would be a service provided to oneself (such as researching an illness at a medical library in the community). ACT5 would be a sustained, personal effort to integrate major life style changes (for example, to become and remain a vegetarian).

When the cl-I-ent featured in the story is an individual or group of individuals (e.g., a family or club), the seven results levels can be described as follows:

ACT1/LEV1 Information is obtained without direct interaction with its provider (e.g., via media)

ACT2/LEV2 Information, brief advice, or some auxiliary service is received through contact (in person, by phone, etc.) with a provider

ACT3/LEV3 A primary service (including counseling or diagnosis) is received through interaction with a provider

MLS4 An indiv-I-dual makes an adjustment in lifestyle or life status that is sustained for more than one month

ACT5/LEV5 A sustained relationship (more than six months) is maintained with a provider that involves multiple services and is intended to empower the indiv-I-dual to move beyond dependency on that relationship

MLS6 An indiv-I-dual sustains an adjustment in lifestyle or life status for more than six months *and* can point to concrete gains in life quality directly related to these changes

MLS7 An indiv-I-dual reaps the full benefits of a lifestyle or life status change as reflected in some truly exceptional performance or contribution (viewed as a lifetime achievement)

When the cl-I-ent featured in a story is a collective (e.g., a task force, an organization, or an institution that is being transformed), the seven results levels can be described in a parallel way:

ACT1/LEV1 Information is obtained without direct interaction with its provider (e.g., via media)

ACT2/LEV2 Information, brief advice, or some auxiliary service is received through contact (in person, by phone, etc.) with a provider

ACT3/LEV3 A primary service (e.g., training or technical assistance) is received through interaction with a provider

MLS4 The un-I-t, organ-I-zation, or inst-I-tution reached a new plateau as demonstrated by its commitment to provide services or take actions that represent a breakthrough for it

ACT5/LEV5 A sustained relationship (more than six months) is maintained with the provider that involves multiple services and is intended to empower the un-I-t, organ-I-zation, or inst-I-tution to move beyond dependency on that relationship

MLS6 The un-I-t, organ-I-zation, or inst-I-tution has provided a service or implemented a program for more than six months that represents a breakthrough for it *and* can show some significant new impacts on the population it served

MLS7 The un-I-t, organ-I-zation, or inst-I-tution has infused the values and spirit of the breakthrough activity into its overall operations *and* has many new types of cl-I-ent impacts at which to point

# STARTING A STORY

As noted earlier, a story is mapped in roughly chronological order beginning with the time that the program first interacted with the cl-I-ent featured in that story. The first map of the story (Map 1) is always a transactional map with program staff (or a staff volunteer) as the change agent. Should there be relevant background information that helps to explain the story, particularly if it justifies the claim of a subsequent cl-I-ent milestone, this material is presented as Map 0 and not scored (i.e., no ACTn or LEVn codes are affixed to the map).

**Map 0**

| STORY ID | PHS-SS | | MAP | 0 | DATE(S) | 3/96 |

| WHO | POP | TYPE | DID WHAT | | LEVEL | MULT |
|---|---|---|---|---|---|---|
| | | | PROGRAM RECEIVED A $25,000 GRANT TO SET UP "PARENTS HELPING PARENTS" PROJECTS IN 4 NEIGHBORHOODS | | | |

| FOR WHOM | POP | TYPE | WITH WHAT RESULT | | LEVEL | MULT |
|---|---|---|---|---|---|---|
| | | | | | | |

| LEVERAGE FRACTION | ACTION POINTS | RECIPIENT POINTS | SELF-DETERMINATION | VILLAGE BUILDING | SERVICES | NETWORKING |
|---|---|---|---|---|---|---|
| | | | | | | |

**Map 1**

| STORY ID | PHS-SS | | MAP | 1 | DATE(S) | |

| WHO | POP | TYPE | DID WHAT | LEVEL | MULT |
|---|---|---|---|---|---|
| TIM AND SUE | 2 | S | RECRUITED PARENTS FROM SOUTHSIDE | ACT2 | 0 |

| FOR WHOM | POP | TYPE | WITH WHAT RESULT | LEVEL | MULT |
|---|---|---|---|---|---|
| PARENTS | 9 | C | AGREED TO SPEARHEAD PROJECT IN THEIR NEIGHBORHOOD | LEV2 | 3 |

| LEVERAGE FRACTION | ACTION POINTS | RECIPIENT POINTS | SELF-DETERMINATION | VILLAGE BUILDING | SERVICES | NETWORKING |
|---|---|---|---|---|---|---|
| 1.0 | 0 | 6 | 0 | 0 | 0 | 6 |

# POPULATION SIZES

Immediately to the right of the spaces on a map where the change agent and recipient are listed are two narrow columns. The first column is used to indicate the *number* of change agents and *number* of recipients featured in this map. However, when the change agent or recipient is a collective (i.e., a team, organization, or institution) acting or reacting as a single entity and not as separate individuals, a population value of 2 is used, by convention, rather than the actual number of people in the group.

Example: Three volunteer staff took turns reading to 14 children at the library's children center. The change agent population is 3; the recipient population is 14.

Example: A funder provided a grant. The population value applied to the funder is 2 and not the number of persons in that organization or serving on the grants committee.

Example: The task force completed an action plan. The population value applied to the task force is 2 and not the number of members on the task force.

Example: The program provided blankets and food to a family of six. The population value applied to the program is 2. However, the population value applied to the family is 6, not 2, since each family member received a share of the food and blankets. They were more akin, here, to six individuals than one family unit.

# POPULATION TYPES

The second column is used to indicate the *type* of change agent and *type* of recipient. In the example above (Map 1), Tim and Sue were two staffers from the program, hence the 2 and S. The nine parents recruited were the cl-I-ents featured in this story, hence the 9 and C.

The following six codes are used to indicate the type of change agent or recipient:

S Program staff
C Cl-I-ent
F Family member of the cl-I-ent
P Individual provider or professional (not staff)
G Group (team, committee, organization, institution, or system)
X Other community member

When a transactional map's change agent has performed the action as a *volunteer*, a "V" is placed before the code. For example, a volunteer organization would be coded as "VG," a doctor providing free medical care would be coded as "VP," and a citizen serving as a volunteer would be coded as "VX." A "volunteer" providing labor is someone receiving no pay or only a portion of normal pay to cover out-of-pocket costs for providing the service. A "volunteer" providing equipment or other non-labor resources is someone doing this free of charge or at a markedly reduced price.

A volunteer from the community who provided a one-time service or short-lived service is coded as "VX." However, if the service was ongoing (e.g., serving as a mentor or care giver) and the program being evaluated provided logistical or other support for the volunteer, then the volunteer is considered surrogate staff and is coded as "VS." This has important implications for leveraging (as discussed in Chapter 6). Furthermore, an individual coded with "VS" can kick off a story (i.e., there is no need to show that person being recruited by the program to serve the cl-I-ent unless this is key to the story).

In the last example, the nine parents recruited had not yet begun functioning as a team, so the population value of 9 was appropriate. However, when six of these parents subsequently planned and implemented a 24-hour child care center in their neighborhood (Map 7 of their story), the code used was G (for group, to indicate they were a team of clients) but the population value assigned was 2 (and not 6), since they were functioning as a team and not as separate individuals. A milestone (MLS4) was applied since this represented a new programming plateau for the community. No recipients as yet benefitted. Later in the story, should it continue, we would expect to see maps with services being provided to children.

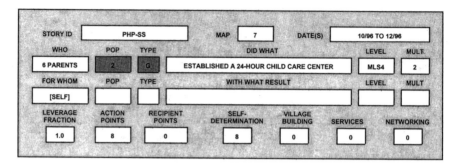

# MAPPING PERSONAL MILESTONES

Since the project, "Parents Helping Parents," was designed to shape the lives of parents so that they could help other parents in their neighborhood, individual plateaus might also be reached in addition to team milestones. For each of these maps, the code C would be used to indicate that it was an individual cl-I-ent of the story that had reached a personal milestone. In addition, each such personal milestone would be mapped separately (i.e., if three cl-I-ents each reached a personal milestone, these would *not* be clumped together on one map but would be documented on three separate maps).

As it turned out, one of the original nine parents—attracted to the possibility of serving as a parish nurse in her community—decided to return to school to pursue a nursing career. She stated that it was her positive experiences working in "Parents Helping Parents" that gave her the confidence and desire to return to school. This major step in her life appeared as Map 11 in the story.

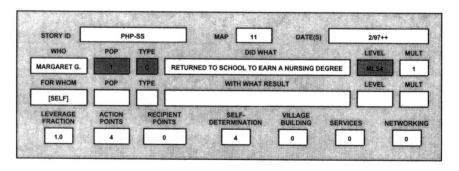

Another parent from the original group began serving as a mentor to a group of three teenagers from her apartment complex. This led to two maps (Maps 12 and 13); the first documenting the volunteer service provided and the second indicating a personal milestone achieved.

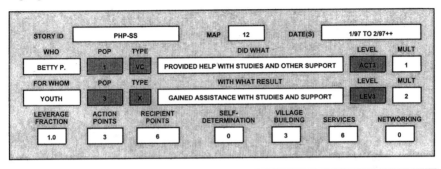

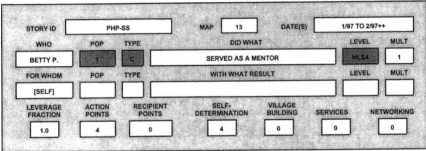

## MAPS COVER THREE-MONTH PERIODS

When a change agent provides *repeated services* during the same three-month period directed at the same cl-I-ent objective, it is mapped only once (with the dates in the Date field that follows the Map Code indicating the time span and the text under Did What noting the frequency as well as type of service provided). However, if the service continued beyond three months, for each additional three-month segment, a new map is added to the story. Thus, for example, a service that is provided continually for a year would result in four maps, one for each three-month period.

To illustrate, in William G.'s story, Ted provided tutoring support for seven months. This led to these three near-identical maps (Maps 1, 2 and 3):

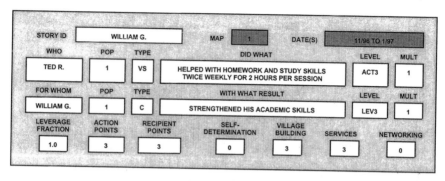

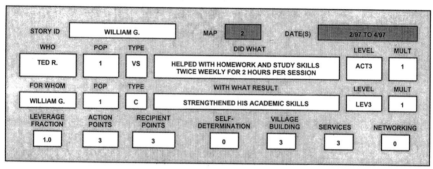

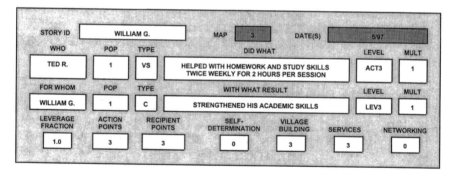

When services are directed at *different* cl-I-ent objectives, then multiple maps are used even when these services occur within the same three-month period. Thus, for example, if program staff provided services to a cl-I-ent aimed at improving the latter's reading skills while also providing services to that ind-I-vidual dealing with some health issue, each set of services would be mapped separately. For either set of services, the three-month rule would apply.

To illustrate, in William G.'s story, program staff supplemented the work of his tutor by taking William on weekend outings during the five-month time period from January 1997 through May 1997. This added two new maps (Maps 4 and 5) to the story.

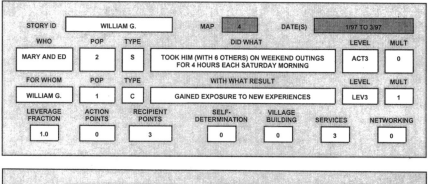

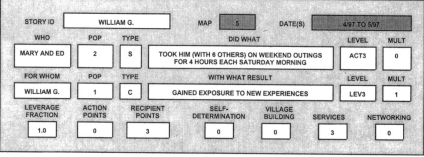

Other examples of the three-month rule:

Example: The program provided space for a support group to meet weekly. The group has met for five months. Two maps would be needed to show the logistical support provided by the program to the support group, one covering the first three months and the second the next two months. (Note: Additional maps would document the actual functioning of the support group.)

Example: The program designed and placed a billboard near the center of town with a strong anti-smoking message aimed at pregnant women. The billboard sign remained there for 13 months and was seen by an average of 2000 persons each month. This would be represented through five maps. The first four would each cover a three-month period; the last would capture the 13th month. The population reached on each of the five maps would be 2000 (or slightly higher), and not 6000, since it would be assumed that roughly the same 2000 persons were seeing the sign again and again.

# HANDOFFS

In many of a program's top stories, it is likely that services will be provided by others in addition to program staff. When the program refers a cl-I-ent or family member to another service provider, the map showing this referral is called a *handoff* and has the program staff as the change agent and the service provider (i.e., the future change agent) as the recipient. This holds true even when direct communications between the two did not occur. So, for example, if the program told a cl-I-ent about a provider, and the cl-I-ent made that contact and received the service, the map describing the referral is still shown as a handoff from the program to the provider. A handoff can be regarded, metaphorically, as the passing of the change agent baton from one entity to another (typically from the program to another service provider).

For handoffs, the *results level is always ACT2/LEV2* and the *recipient population for the handoff is always "1."* This convention was introduced to avoid over-scoring the impact of a handoff. For example, if a clinic received a referral and then provided a service for a fee; without this convention, the referral would earn more points than the service provided. In the next example, where the program made a handoff to a clinic that provided charity care through volunteers, the population in Map 2 is "1" even though this was an organization that otherwise would carry a population of "2." However, in the paired map (Map 3), when the organization is the change agent, a population of "2" is applied.

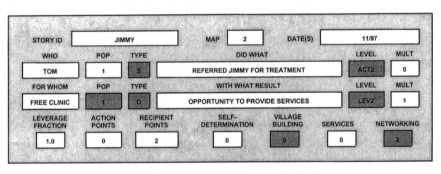

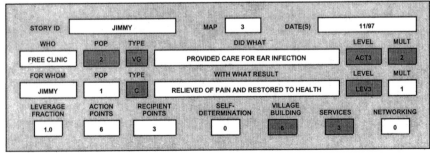

Sets of related maps are used to document *assisted handoffs*. These are cases when either or both of the following two situations arise: (1) the cl-I-ent took unusual steps—for him or her—to follow through on the referral by the program to the second agency and/or (2) the program staff provided one or more auxiliary services (e.g., transportation or child care) to allow the cl-I-ent to follow through. By convention, *auxiliary services are coded as ACT2/LEV2* and not as ACT3/ LEV3, as they would be if they were primary services. Similarly, the unusual steps taken by the cl-I-ent are coded as ACT2 (self-determination) and not as MLS4, since they represent one-time efforts and not a sustained change in life style or status lasting for more than one month.

To illustrate, consider Tanya's story:

Tanya is 19 years old and the mother of two young girls. She is single and lives with her maternal grandmother in a three-bedroom apartment in Prince George's County, Maryland. She has never had or even applied for a job, apart from raising the girls and helping out in the apartment. The program, New Start, has provided Tanya with basic work skills training, introduced her to computer data entry, and assisted her in finding affordable child care (for the hours her grandmother is at work). She is about to go on her first job interview, which has been arranged by the program, and she is very nervous. Peggy, her mentor at New Start, rehearses the interview process with her several times and assures her that not getting this particular job is not the end of the world. Peggy drives Tanya to the interview and waits for her in the parking lot. An hour later, Tanya reappears with a big grin on her face. She starts work the next day.

The four maps of Tanya's story (Maps 6–9) that cover the job referral and successful interview would appear as follows:

| STORY ID | TANYA | | MAP | 6 | DATE(S) | | 10/97 | |
|---|---|---|---|---|---|---|---|---|
| **WHO** | **POP** | **TYPE** | | **DID WHAT** | | | **LEVEL** | **MULT** |
| PEGGY | 1 | S | | ARRANGED JOB INTERVIEW | | | ACT2 | 0 |
| **FOR WHOM** | **POP** | **TYPE** | | **WITH WHAT RESULT** | | | **LEVEL** | **MULT** |
| ABC CORP | 1 | G | | HAS JOB CANDIDATE TO INTERVIEW | | | LEV2 | 1 |
| **LEVERAGE FRACTION** | **ACTION POINTS** | **RECIPIENT POINTS** | | **SELF-DETERMINATION** | **VILLAGE BUILDING** | **SERVICES** | **NETWORKING** | |
| 1.0 | 0 | 2 | | 0 | 0 | 0 | 2 | |

| STORY ID | TANYA | | MAP | 7 | DATE(S) | 10/97 | |
|---|---|---|---|---|---|---|---|
| WHO | POP | TYPE | DID WHAT | | | LEVEL | MULT |
| PEGGY | 1 | S | PROVIDED TRANSPORTATION FOR INTERVIEW | | | ACT2 | 0 |
| FOR WHOM | POP | TYPE | WITH WHAT RESULT | | | LEVEL | MULT |
| TANYA | 1 | C | ABLE TO KEEP APPOINTMENT | | | LEV2 | 1 |
| LEVERAGE FRACTION | ACTION POINTS | RECIPIENT POINTS | SELF-DETERMINATION | VILLAGE BUILDING | SERVICES | NETWORKING | |
| 1.0 | 0 | 2 | 0 | 0 | 2 | 0 | |

| STORY ID | TANYA | | MAP | 8 | DATE(S) | 10/97 | |
|---|---|---|---|---|---|---|---|
| WHO | POP | TYPE | DID WHAT | | | LEVEL | MULT |
| TANYA | 1 | C | OVERCAME FEAR AND WENT ON FIRST INTERVIEW | | | ACT2 | 1 |
| FOR WHOM | POP | TYPE | WITH WHAT RESULT | | | LEVEL | MULT |
| [SELF] | | | | | | | |
| LEVERAGE FRACTION | ACTION POINTS | RECIPIENT POINTS | SELF-DETERMINATION | VILLAGE BUILDING | SERVICES | NETWORKING | |
| 1.0 | 2 | 0 | 2 | 0 | 0 | 0 | |

| STORY ID | TANYA | | MAP | 9 | DATE(S) | 10/97 | |
|---|---|---|---|---|---|---|---|
| WHO | POP | TYPE | DID WHAT | | | LEVEL | MULT |
| ABC CORP | 2 | G | OFFERED A JOB | | | ACT3 | 0 |
| FOR WHOM | POP | TYPE | WITH WHAT RESULT | | | LEVEL | MULT |
| TANYA | 1 | C | GOT HER FIRST EVER JOB | | | LEV3 | 1 |
| LEVERAGE FRACTION | ACTION POINTS | RECIPIENT POINTS | SELF-DETERMINATION | VILLAGE BUILDING | SERVICES | NETWORKING | |
| 1.0 | 0 | 3 | 0 | 0 | 3 | 0 | |

Should Tanya remain on the job for more than one month, a milestone (MLS4) would certainly be warranted. This would appear as a new map in the story.

Handoffs that do not lead to follow-through services are not typically mapped. Thus, in the above example, if ABC Corp. did not offer Tanya the job, Maps 6–9 would not appear in Tanya's story. The logic here is that each map of a story represents some direct or indirect gain for the cl-I-ent. A handoff that does not lead anywhere would normally not be considered a gain. There are exceptions to this rule. It might be argued, for example, that the first job interview was a gain for Tanya (i.e., an experience with future value) even if it did not result in a job. In such cases, maps would be included in the story related to the handoff.

# ACCOUNTING FOR DURATION

As noted earlier, a MLS4 represents a shift toward a positive behavior that is sustained for more than one month. A MLS4 is not assigned for a single short-lived event, regardless of how dramatic it is. To illustrate, a cl-I-ent's decision to stop using drugs would alone not be enough to warrant a milestone. A milestone would be assigned to the cl-I-ent's story only after more than a month of drug-free behavior was demonstrated.

A MLS6 is a shift in lifestyle that is maintained for more than six months. It must be preceded by maps indicating both a MLS4 achievement and cl-I-ent activity at Level 5. This activity can involve a coach, mentor, or support group; or it can be self-directed by the cl-I-ent. However, in the latter case, no points for the MLS6 would be awarded to the program (since, as explained in Chapter 6, the leverage fraction would be 0).

The ACT5→LEV5 relationship is reached only after six months of sustained interaction between change agent and recipient. Therefore, in mapping such a relationship, the map at Level 5 must be preceded by at least two maps (each covering three months) showing an ACT3→LEV3 relationship between the same parties, as well as a MLS4 indicating growth in the recipient.

> **Example:** A retired schoolteacher agreed to serve as a mentor for a third grader who was having academic and personal difficulties at school. The mentoring relationship began in October 1997 and continued through May 1998. At least four maps would be required to show the relationship. Map 1 would cover the period from October through December and be coded as ACT3→LEV3. Map 2 would be similarly coded for the period from January through March. Map 3 would be a milestone for the child at MLS4. Map 4 would cover the period from April through May and be coded as an ACT5→LEV5 relationship.

The six-month rule is a necessary, but not sufficient, condition for an ACT5→LEV5 relationship. As discussed in Chapter 3, there must also be "intimacy" between the change agent and recipient reflected in multiple services, warm-hearted give and take, and gradual shifting of the locus of control from the change agent to the recipient. A single service relationship (e.g., an agency providing transportation or food services to the cl-I-ent) would not be elevated to a Level 5 relationship even after six months had passed.

# ONLY ACTIVITIES DURING THE PAST TWO YEARS ARE SCORED

Evaluations typically run on an annual cycle, established by the funder. In contrast, stories unfold according to their own natural rhythm and may cross evaluation cycles and take months or years to play out. Thus, when mapping a story, it may be necessary to go back two years or longer to capture the full extent of program involvement with the cl-I-ent. Consequently, it is common for stories to run into a second, third, or even fourth evaluation cycle.

By convention, when scoring stories of long duration, only maps with dates of two years or less from the cutoff date for the evaluation report are scored. The earlier maps are zeroed out (i.e., included in the story to provide context but not scored). This allows the entire story to be told, but avoids crediting a program for work that was done well before the current evaluation cycle. So, for example, if an evaluation began in January 1998 and the first annual report was due a year later (January 1999), the program stories in that report might go back as far as the early 1990's but only maps with dates between January 1997 and December 1998 would be scored and included in the analysis of the program.

Results Mapping can be applied at any time to ongoing programs to capture how successful they have been with their top stories during the most recent years. One does not have to design an evaluation plan; one just starts mapping. For this reason, Results Mapping is ideal for programs with little or no evaluation budgets that still want to benefit from the rich feedback that a comprehensive evaluation can provide. Mapping can also be appended to ongoing evaluations using more conventional methods (e.g., multi-year, quasi-experimental evaluation designs) to supplement and enrich these efforts.

For start-up programs, it may take six months or more before the program has sufficient impact on its cl-I-ents so that its best work can be distinguished from more "average" activity. We recommend that a start-up program begin thinking from the outset about the types of information that will be needed to relate and map its best stories, and set up an information system or case notes format that will facilitate later story mapping. Such a system would need to capture all key program services provided to the cl-I-ent (in three-month blocks), all referrals that led to needed services, all cl-I-ent milestones linked to the program's contributions, and all associated cl-I-ent actions to assist others.

As suggested in the previous chapter, a first-year evaluation based on Results Mapping should include a program's 12 to 15 top cl-I-ent stories. In the second and subsequent years of the evaluation, we suggest increasing that number to 25 to 30 stories. At any time, new maps can be added to a story. Therefore, a story featuring the same cl-I-ent may have a different point value (referred to as its *story score*) from one evaluation to the next. Since only the last two years' worth of point productivity will be included in the analysis, some stories likely will be dropped each round and replaced with others where the program has made greater contributions in recent years. However, for programs whose cl-I-ents are ne-I-ghborhoods, organ-I-zations, or inst-I-tutions, there may not be many total stories to tell. In these situations, all stories should be mapped and included in the analysis—but, again, only scored for the last two years.

# COMPARABLE CL-I-ENTS

One final note. Only comparable stories can be included in an analysis. If the program has two or more distinctly different types of cl-I-ents, then requirements for Results Mapping are 12 to 15 top stories per cl-I-ent type. To illustrate, in our current evaluation of family resource centers in Cincinnati, each of the five centers included in the study provides services to individuals and families *but also* spearheads community development projects. For the baseline for this evaluation, each center provided its 15 top service-based stories *and* its 15 top community development stories. In the second year of the evaluation, these numbers were increased to 30 top service-based stories and 30 top community development stories. As a variation on this last point, should program management want to contrast the work of different staff or teams that are working with similar cl-I-ents, it will also need 12 to 15 top stories per staff member/team to allow useful analysis.

# QUIZ 4

4.1. When would a story be split into two or more separate stories?

4.2. What change agent type (S or VS) would be assigned to a teenager who worked for the program during the summer and was paid minimum wage?

4.3. What change agent type (S or VS) would be assigned to a teenager who worked for the program for two months to satisfy her school's community service requirement?

4.4. How many maps would be included in a story to show that a cl-I-ent attended weekly support group meetings for four months?

4.5. A program's best story dated back to 1993, but is ongoing (i.e., services are still being provided to the featured cl-I-ent). When it maps that story and computes its score, is it possible that the story will not score very high? If so, is something wrong with the scoring system?

# What the Mapped Data Show

*We often tend to limit our explorations of what's possible by
surrounding ourselves with large amounts of information that
tell us nothing new. We collect information from measures
that tell us how we are doing—whether we're up to standard,
whether we're meeting our goals. But these measures...keep
us distracted from questioning our experience in a way that
could create greater possibilities. They don't ask us to question why we're doing what we're doing. They don't ask us to
notice what learning is available from all those things we decided not to measure (Wheatley & Kellner-Rogers, 1996,
p. 26).*

**TURNING ANECDOTES INTO "HARD DATA"**

**Best Program Work is Documented**
- **Narrative Accounts**
- **Mapped Stories**

**Outcome Data are Provided**
- LEV3 interim outcomes
- MLS4 intermediate outcomes
- MLS6 longer-term outcomes
- MLS7 ultimate outcomes

**Performance Measures are Available**
- **Overall Point Production**
- **Services by Level and Provider Type**
- **Village Building/Networking Activity**

Mapped stories afford a wealth of information regarding what a program does best. The stories themselves are illuminating. It is remarkable how few persons actually know how a program works to get its top results. Few Board members, program administrators, funders, or even co-workers can relate in any detail the twists and turns of stories involving a program's most successful cl-I-ents—beyond perhaps its first two "super success" stories. The 12 to 15 stories compiled in each mapping cycle for analysis often represent the first comprehensive picture of the day-to-day performance of the program ever captured. The data these stories yield make it clear how the program works to achieve its successes *and* where it needs to work harder or more effectively to achieve more of these.

Few social, health, and prevention programs are as potent and effective as they can be. The best programs can get better and the more average programs have far to go in optimizing their resources and services on behalf of their cl-I-ents. And one key to such dramatic improvement involves learning from their best work: making today's positive exceptions tomorrow's norms.

Through Results Mapping we can address a fundamental evaluation question: *To what degree is the program living up to its potential?* This is a question not often asked. Most evaluations tend to focus on a less ambitious question: *Is the program meeting its promised targets?* Although that is a good question, by tracking a program's contributions toward cl-I-ent outcomes, we are able to answer it while probing deeper.

Strong programs appreciate this deeper level of inquiry because they know they are good at what they do, would like others to recognize this, and want to get even better. These programs have no problems in meeting targets and typically learn little from evaluation findings that simply report this fact. Their administrators and staff tend to view evaluation data as something to be prepared for others but of little relevance for day-to-day operations.

We are discovering that weaker programs, while suspicious and somewhat skeptical at first, also quickly learn to like this deeper question. The answers provided through Results Mapping make it easy to pinpoint program shortfalls (e.g., the absence of timely follow-through with cl-I-ents or lack of attention to the role that volunteers might play) and direct managers and staff to actions that strengthen what they do. With a focus on continual program improvement, programs more easily meet stated targets, look good to their funders, and move up in the rankings toward the performance levels of strong programs. Although I frequently hear programs complain that they shouldn't be compared with other programs—since they are unique—they do recognize the value in comparing their own performance patterns from one evaluation period to the next.

How far is a program from reaching its potential? The answer begins to reveal itself when scores from a program's 12 to 15 top stories are plotted in descending order. One of four profiles results. Programs with the first profile (Figure 5.1) each have one or two anecdotes that are truly exceptional for them (and have

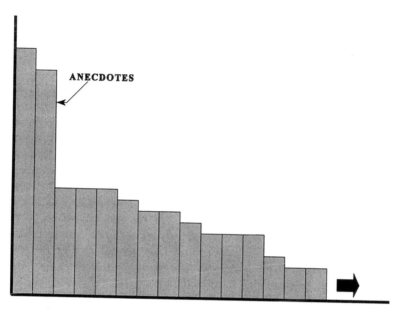

Figure 5.1. Profile of "fix it" type program with anecdotes. Beyond the first two stories, the contributions of the program are modest and similar.

story scores far higher than the rest). Beyond these, the program's "best stories" are rather average. The anecdotes must be viewed as anomalies. The evidence does not suggest that the programs can reproduce these levels of success with other cl-I-ents. They are far from their potential.

In the next profile (Figure 5.2), the programs show more promise. In addition to their high-scoring anecdotes, the programs have a second set of stories that score well above their more average stories. The programs seem to have figured out what it takes to make strong contributions to cl-I-ents, although still not consistently nor frequently.

The third profile (Figure 5.3) is associated with a set of programs that are applying best practices across the high end of their cl-I-ent base. However, the drop from story to story is a bit severe. Based on limited evidence, I have posited that a truly high-performing program will have no more than a threefold decline from its top to its 15th best story. Thus, the programs matching this third profile need to apply their best practices more frequently with their cl-I-ents to push up the entire set of scores.

The fourth profile (Figure 5.4) is rare. Programs matching this profile are consistently applying best practices to achieve high scores across their top stories. Their top stories earn a lot of points (comparable to, or considerably higher than,

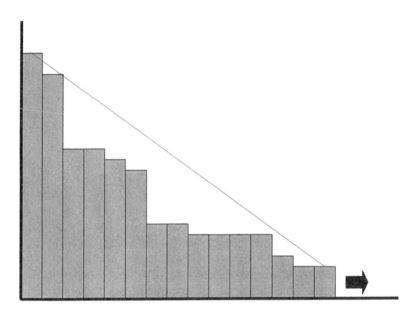

Figure 5.2. Profile of a program with a modest degree of success. The blank space below the dotted line suggests room for further improvement.

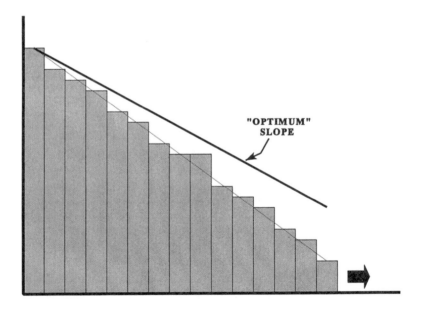

Figure 5.3. Profile of programs consistently applying best practices. The drop from story to story, however, is severe.

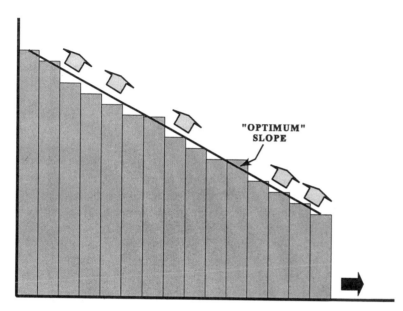

"OPTIMUM"
SLOPE

Figure 5.4. Profile of an optimum program. Its challenge is to push the envelope even further across its entire cl-I-ent base.

the scores for the exceptional anecdotes in the first profile) and the decline from story to story is relatively slow. These programs may be operating at or near peak performance. However, it is possible that some of them can ratchet up all their scores by introducing some new element to their mix of activities *and* increase the total number of cl-I-ents served.

To improve quality and advance toward excellence, one must unsettle those who maintain the status quo. This holds for science, for art, for success in business, for shared beliefs and prejudices, and for programs. Head counts, satisfaction survey results, and bottom-line measures of outcome and efficiency—the standard feedback to date of program evaluations—are rarely unsettling. These data do not often provoke or promote fundamental change. When positive, they merely reinforce the status quo; when negative, they become the points from which to attack the logic or practices of the evaluators.

Results Mapping provides feedback with an unsettling punch. We do this out of appreciation (for what the programs can contribute to their cl-I-ents and society), and not out of malice or to be mischievous. In a very commonsensical way, the approach is used to uncover for scrutiny the very best work of a program— work of which line staff and managers ought to be proud. If that work is truly superior, it scores high and graphs well. If there are gaps or inconsistencies in performance, these are reflected through the data generated. "Here are your scores," we say. "What do you think of them? Are there findings that are disturbing or a source of concern? If so, let's talk about what might be changed in the program to move the program closer to where you wish it to be!"

To be unsettling, we document through Results Mapping how much the program is contributing toward outcomes. We examine its top stories and ask:

*In how many of these stories has a cl-I-ent reached MLS6?* What did it take to get there? What outstanding or perceptive actions did the program staff take? Are there enough of these longer-term outcomes appearing in the top stories?

*And what about MLS4s?* There may be a lot of these, but is there a pattern? Do certain combinations of staff-led actions produce more such milestones? What do the more successful cl-I-ents share in terms of characteristics, contexts, and needs from the program? Are you confident that you can contribute to more of these milestones during the next round of the evaluation?

To be unsettling, we focus on how effective the program has been in networking with other service providers in the community. We examine the networking points from story to story and see where these partnerships have been most successful in moving cl-I-ents to milestones. And ask:

*Has there been enough networking?* How often were cl-I-ents directed to all the services they needed and in a timely manner?

*What are new networking options that might be tapped in the next round?* What steps have to be taken during the next evaluation cycle to exploit these options in support of a cl-I-ent's total needs?

To be unsettling, we focus on activities with volunteers. We array the points earned by different types of volunteers. We determine the extent to which programs have made creative use of their cl-I-ents as helpers for others or made it more likely that they would be positioned to be helpful to others in the future. We then ask:

*Are your staff doing too much?* Aren't there activities that might better be turned over to cl-I-ents and volunteers?

*How frequently have your cl-I-ents been provided with opportunities to be helpful to others—one important key to growth and health?* Can more of these opportunities be made available during the next evaluation cycle?

We are particularly unsettling when we provide scores to programs and especially to funders. There is something about a score that provokes an emotional reaction—likely a throwback to school days. And, unfortunately, a score is still viewed as "harder evidence" than a story. While physicists and other leading edge scientists now recognize that quality is more substantial than quantity, most of the rest of us still believe the opposite. And I, for one, while promoting the use of a mix of evaluation data, am not opposed to scores being part of that mix. I enjoy following sports and recognize the critical function that scores and other performance measures play in pushing athletes to their current limits and beyond. I am also a fan of total quality management and its guiding principle: *Only what gets measured gets attention; only what gets attention gets fixed.*

The blending of stories, outcome data, *and* scores yields the "hard data" that are needed for fair and comprehensive evaluations of programs engaged in healing, transformation, and prevention. "Hard data," to me, are those that (1) are accurate, (2) provide the kinds of evidence that evoke confidence among decision-makers *and* (3) are consistent with the best *current* science from those fields in which the latest truths and insights regarding human nature are being generated.

The "hard data" provided through Results Mapping are useful to funders engaged in outcome-based funding. With clear documentation in hand of what programs have been able to accomplish with their best cl-I-ents, and with data to estimate how much the *overall program* has been contributing toward making future cl-I-ent transformations more likely, funders are better positioned to make realistic demands on these and similar programs. It becomes possible, for example, to negotiate performance-based contracts where, under terms acceptable to both funder and program, reimbursements can be linked to progress of cl-I-ents (e.g., numbers reaching MLS4 and MLS6) and associated point productivity (to reward, where appropriate, increases in village building and networking activity).[1]

When similar programs are funded in different sites, Results Mapping data from each site can be contrasted. Since programs may be serving different population mixes and have differing conditions and constraints under which they operate, contrasts and comparisons must be made with caution. Still, much can be learned by contrasting the top stories and associated practices of different programs. Funders and others can use the stories and associated data to explore with programs why there are cross-program differences. And, having accounted for site-to-site variations, funders might reasonably ask why they should continue to fund sites that are far less productive or that are less committed than others in contributing to cl-I-ent progress.

[1] Currently, Results Mapping scores are presented as points. In the next generation of the approach, we expect to be able to translate story data into social cost savings, expressed in dollars or units of credit. This will permit return-on-investment calculations to be made, as a further aid to program and funder decision-making.

We urge programs using Results Mapping to join our informal learning network. We continue to learn new things about this relatively new approach that we are happy to share with others. This book is a first step in this direction. We have set up a web site (www.pire.org.results_mapping) that readers are encouraged to visit from time to time to discover what we are currently up to.

We are anxious for the approach to be applied and gain acceptance across the country. But we are also concerned about quality control. We would hate for Results Mapping to gain a bad reputation through misuse. For this reason, we protect the term legally and require active permission or formal licensing agreements for the proprietary aspects of the product. Naturally, we also want to be kept informed of Results Mapping applications and be called on to answer questions or to troubleshoot where needed. And we are, of course, pleased to be invited to participate in new adventures. So keep in touch.[2]

# QUIZ 5

5.1. What are likely causes of staff frustration or concern when they first start capturing their top stories using Results Mapping? What might be done to reduce or eliminate these?

5.2. What program actions are most likely to lead to increases in points during the first months of using Results Mapping? What actions are most likely to lead to these increases after five to six months? What about after a year?

5.3. What arguments would you use to gain support for Results Mapping from a key stakeholder (funder or political leader) who feels pressured to show that funds being spent are making a *real difference* in the community?

---

[2] We can be reached at The Results Mapping Laboratory, Pacific Institute for Research and Evaluation, 121 West Rosemary, Second Floor, Chapel Hill, NC 27516.

# II

# Practice

# 6

# How to Score a Results Map

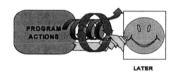

LATER

☞ **MULTIPLICITY OF SERVICES AND OUTCOMES**

☞ **CASE MANAGEMENT/WRAPAROUND**

☞ **NETWORKING/VILLAGE BUILDING**

☞ **ASSET-FOCUSED/PREVENTION-ORIENTED**

☞ **OUTSIDE INFLUENCES ("OPEN SYSTEM")**

☞ **SELF-DETERMINATION/EMPOWERMENT**

A number of characteristics separate programs engaged in healing and transformation from the "fix it/cure it" types. First and foremost, they *contribute* to the likelihood of long-term outcomes rather than primarily *produce* shorter-term outcomes. In doing so, they typically provide a range of services aimed at a range of interim and intermediate outcomes key to longer-term success.

Second, responses to cl-I-ents tend to vary across their cl-I-ents. A staff person is typically assigned to serve as the case manager to coordinate these services. For complex cases, teams may be formed that include the case manager, the cl-I-ent (where possible), family members, other key professionals, and community support persons (e.g., clergy or youth club director). The teams meet regularly to develop, implement, and update a "wraparound" plan designed to meet the unique needs of the cl-I-ent in multiple domains (e.g., mental health, physical health, housing, education, and spiritual).

Third, these programs seldom are the only service provider. More frequently, they network with other programs, through referrals and collaborations, to maximize use of the resources that are available in the community to serve the needs of their cl-I-ents. Since these programs are typically under-funded given the demand for services, they rely on "volunteer power" to augment and complement staff resources. But it goes deeper. The philosophy underlying many of these programs is that "it takes a village to raise a cl-I-ent." The generosity, love, attention, and support freely given by volunteers may sometimes be the "Factor X" that sparks growth or spontaneous healing. The power of community has long been recognized. As urban planning students in the 1960s, my peers and I were greatly influenced by the classic *The Death and Life of Great American Cities* (Jacobs, 1961). Rekindling the spirit of community is essential to re-inventing American society, and healing and transformation programs are a leading edge in this communitarian movement (Etzioni, 1993).

Fourth, there is an emerging trend in prevention and related youth development fields, also evident in forward-thinking service providers, to approach cl-I-ents through their assets rather than deficits. Rather than focusing on warning messages, laws, and controlled environments to keep youth in line, programs are challenging and assisting youth to be *creative* and *responsible*. This demands that program staff approach their work with open-mindedness, trust in others, and an adventurous spirit—qualities not often associated with fix it/cure it programs.

Fifth, because of their long-term view, programs engaged in healing and transformation remain open to new opportunities and threats that may dramatically alter the range and types of services they offer to their cl-I-ents.

Sixth, and probably most important, these programs not only focus on the ability of their cl-I-ents to take responsibility for their own growth and healing, they depend on it for success. In so doing, they are tapping into an inherent human trait—the need to grow. Life is about growth and change; many problems in society can be linked to the inability or denial of the opportunity to participate fully in the growth and prosperity of society. And growth is twofold:

A person must grow as well as help grow. He must grow inwardly through the contributions of others, as well as outwardly by his own contributions. Unfortunately, this fact of natural life has often not been recognized nor understood (Land, 1973, p. 126).

Results Mapping has been designed to capture, in a methodical and informative manner, the ways these six characteristics play out in programs engaged in healing, transformation, and prevention. The use of mapped stories seems, to me, to be critical to the ability to accomplish this, as is the ability to score and rate the programs based on the levels of service, networking, village building, and cl-I-ent growth and progress evident in their top stories.

# TYPES OF POINTS

Here is how the scoring works. Each map of a story (other than background maps and maps documenting accomplishments prior to the two-year evaluation period) can earn the program either action points or recipient points, and sometimes both.

**Action points** are awarded to the program whenever a change agent takes action for self-benefit or community-benefit (i.e., when it is a self-referential map) *or* when the change agent is functioning as a volunteer/village builder (and the change agent type is VS, VC, VF, VP, VG, or VX). These latter action points are bonuses for the program to acknowledge its ability to encourage the growth of its cl-I-ents or to mobilize volunteers as "village builders." When the change agent of a map is a paid staff member of the program or of another agency, or anyone else who is receiving fair compensation for the services offered, no action points are earned (but recipient points *are* earned).

**Recipient points** are awarded whenever there is a recipient (i.e., for all transactional maps where the population being reached is not zero). A recipient population of zero is a special case. It is used when the change agent has made a contribution toward a community service (i.e., an ACT3 for multiple recipients) but is not the direct service provider (i.e., there is no direct contact between the change agent and the population who will benefit from the actions taken). An example would be a group of youth who helped clean up a park. This convention was applied in Map 6 of Frances's story in Chapter 3, where she was helping to prepare meals for home delivery.

Action and recipient points are tallied map by map. The sum of the action points and recipient points for a map is referred to as the *map score*. The sum of these points across all maps in the story is the *story score*.

| STORY ID | | | | MAP | | DATE(S) | | |
|---|---|---|---|---|---|---|---|---|
| WHO | POP | TYPE | DID WHAT | | | | LEVEL | MULT |
| | | | | | | | | |
| FOR WHOM | POP | TYPE | WITH WHAT RESULT | | | | LEVEL | MULT |
| | | | | | | | | |
| LEVERAGE FRACTION | ACTION POINTS | RECIPIENT POINTS | SELF-DETERMINATION | VILLAGE BUILDING | SERVICES | NETWORKING | | |
| | | | | | | | | |

The terms *action points* and *recipient points* do not convey as much as we might like back to programs and funders. To remedy this:

- Action points from self-referential maps are referred to as *self-determination points*.
- Action points from transactional maps are also called *village-building points*.
- Recipient points are also termed *service points* or, for handoffs, *networking points*.

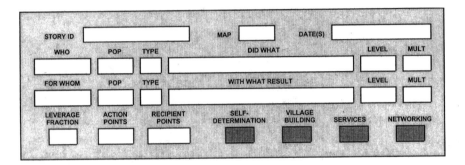

# SCORING ALGORITHM

Computing the action points is similar to computing the recipient points. In both cases, the calculation involves multiplying the results level by a population multiplier and by a map leverage fraction. These two new concepts (the population multiplier and leverage fraction) will first be discussed; then the scoring will be illustrated using the examples from earlier chapters.

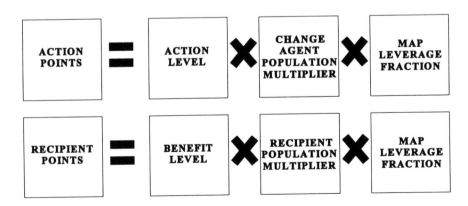

## THE POPULATION MULTIPLIER

Population multipliers are used whenever multiple change agents or multiple recipients are involved in the transaction being mapped. These multipliers serve to minimize point distortions when large numbers of persons are involved in low-level activities (e.g., 3000 persons receiving health tips in the mail or 200 persons attending a rally). The use of these multipliers can also be justified on theoretical grounds. Social impact theory, for example, suggests that the impact of a message on recipients decreases as the size of the target audience increases. And experienced trainers will readily admit that they are more effective in small-group settings (where there can be more give-and-take with trainees) than in auditorium-like settings.

A quasi-logarithmic scale is used to convert the actual number of change agents or recipients to a corresponding population multiplier (Table 6.1). A logarithmic scale would get to 10,001+ in six steps, rather than the ten in the table, and would not allow sufficient differentiation between small and medium sized groups who are the subjects of most of the stories featuring multi-person cl-I-ents (e.g., families or youth groups).

As can be seen in Table 6.1, the population multipliers range in value from 1 through 10. A multiplier of 1 is used when there is a single recipient or change agent. A multiplier of 2 is used when there are 2 to 5 recipients or 2 to 5 change agents. The highest population multiplier is used when there are more than 10,000 recipients (which typically would occur for low results levels). This scoring convention essentially equates—for program scoring purposes—a very low-level result (scored as 1 point) reaching 51 to 100 people (hence, a 6-point multiplier) to a long-term outcome (i.e, a milestone 6) being attained by a single person. Other conventions might have been used, but this one is easy to apply and leads to story scores with good face validity (i.e., programs or funders reviewing any two maps will most always agree that the one earning more points deserves the higher score

**Table 6.1.** Population Multiplier Conversion Table[a]

| Actual number | Population multiplier | Actual number | Population multiplier |
|---|---|---|---|
| 1 | 1 | 51–100 | 6 |
| 2–5 | 2 | 101–500 | 7 |
| 6–10 | 3 | 501–1,000 | 8 |
| 11–25 | 4 | 1,001–10,000 | 9 |
| 26–50 | 5 | 10,001+ | 10 |

[a]The actual number of change agents or recipients is matched with the multiplier (e.g., 12 is matched with 4; 120 with 7).

based on the program's relative impact on the recipients appearing in these maps).

To illustrate the effects of the multiplier, how many points should a program earn for a mass mailing providing some health or prevention information? The results level assigned to "received information through a mass mailing" would be ACT1→LEV1 (with a benefit level of 1). If 10,000 persons were reached, we wouldn't want the score for the benefit to be 1 × 10,000 = 10,000 recipient points. This would bring us to head counts as a principal factor in establishing program productivity and, if used to rate program performance, might encourage programs to concentrate on low-level benefits that reach large numbers rather than on more quality-rich activities that reach far fewer persons and are harder to implement. Instead, for the example above, we apply a population multiplier of 9 to the raw score of 1, resulting in 1 × 9 = 9 recipient points.

Similarly, if 16 youth are trained as a group, this is different from each receiving personal training on a one-on-one basis. Using the population multiplier, the group training for the 16 youth (ACT3→LEV3) would earn the program 3 × 4 = 12 recipient points and not 3 × 16 = 48 recipient points. Continuing this example, should two staff volunteers conduct this training, the additional action points earned by the program would be 3 × 2 = 6 action (village-building) points. Should there be three staff volunteers conducting the training, there would still be 3 × 2 = 6 action points earned since the multiplier is the same for two or three change agents. It would take six to ten staff volunteers to increase the action points to 3 × 3 = 9.

# EXCEPTIONS WHEN DETERMINING THE POPULATION MULTIPLIER

There are a few cases in which conventions rather than the conversion table are used to determine the population multiplier.

First, for transactional maps, when change agents are *not* volunteers, the population multiplier assigned to the *change agent portion* of the map is 0. This ensures that bonus points for village building are not earned for this activity. As a simple check, if the code for the change agent type begins with a "V" (e.g., VS or VG or VX), then use the conversion table to determine the population multiplier for the change agents; otherwise, assign a "0" to that value.

Second, as introduced in Chapter 4, when the change agent or recipient of a map is a collective (coded as "G"), the *population* assigned to that entity is "2"—as is the population multiplier. This convention applies to task forces, clinics, coalitions, funding groups, schools, and other aggregates; its use stresses that the collective is functioning as a single entity and not as a collection of separate individuals.

There are two exceptions to the population = 2 rule, however, when mapping entities:

- When this entity is operating as the change agent of a map, and there is no "V" in the code indicating that the entity is serving in a volunteer capacity, the *population multiplier* assigned is "0" to avoid crediting village building points.
- When the entity is the recipient of a handoff (rather than being provided with some direct service), the *population* assigned to the map, as well as the *population multiplier*, is "1" and not "2."

# THE MAP LEVERAGE FRACTION

This fraction is applied to reduce points earned by the program when the actions taken and results achieved are well beyond those that can reasonably be attributed *in full* to previous actions of program staff or staff volunteers. There are two cases in which this applies:

Case 1.  When the map's change agent has not been in direct contact with program staff or staff volunteers or the subject of a handoff from the staff.

Case 2.  When the level of action or milestone reached on the map is two or more results levels higher than any previous actions taken by staff or staff volunteers to encourage this result.

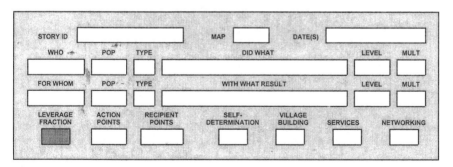

To determine the fraction, we observe who is the map's change agent. If the change agent is a program staffer or staff volunteer, the fraction is automatically assigned a value of "1." If the change agent is not staff, two tests are used to determine the leverage fraction. First, how far separated is the change agent from any program staffer in a related map? If there is one degree of separation (i.e., there was either direct contact between any staffer and this change agent or a handoff between the two in some earlier map), the leverage fraction remains at "1." If there are two degrees of separation (i.e., the connection between any staffer and this change agent is through some intermediate change agent), the leverage fraction becomes "0.5" and half credit is earned by the program for the accomplishments on this map. If there are more than two degrees of separation, the leverage fraction becomes "0" and no credit is earned by the program for the accomplishments on this map.

Example: John, a staffer, taught a relaxation technique to Mary, a cl-I-ent. Mary, in turn, taught the technique to her son. The leverage fraction for the transaction between Mary and her son would be 1.0 since Mary (the change agent of this map) had been in direct contact with the program (via John). However, if Mary's son were to share the technique with schoolmates, a leverage fraction of 0.5 would be applied. In this case, there would have been no direct contact between the map's change agent (i.e., the son) and the program.

The second test is applied if the leverage fraction is not already "0" based on the first test. The results level of the map is compared to the highest results level of a previous, *related* map where a staffer was the change agent. If the results level of the current map is lower, the same as, or one level higher than the level of that staff map, the leverage fraction does not change. If the results level of the current map is two levels higher than the staff map, the leverage fraction remains or is changed to "0.5." If the results level of the current map is three or more levels higher than the staff map, the leverage fraction is changed to "0."

Example: John, a staffer, taught a relaxation technique to Mary, a cl-I-ent. This was an ACT3→LEV3 transaction. Mary began practicing the technique on a regular basis and, after two months, her stress level was reduced dramatically. This was a MLS4 for which the program earned full credit (since Level 4 is one level higher than Level 3, the highest level at which the program provided related services to her). Based on her positive experience, Mary signed up for yoga classes. This was an ACT3 for which the program also earned full credit. During the next six months, Mary completely changed her lifestyle and became a practicing Buddhist. She was now operating at Level 5 and earned a personal MLS6. The program received half credit for the Level 5 activity (since it was two levels higher than the highest action level of the program) but no credit for the new milestone (since it was three levels higher).

# EXAMPLES OF SCORING

Examples from earlier chapters will next be used to illustrate the scoring algorithm. In all cases, the map leverage fraction was 1.0. In the more complex cases presented in the next chapter, several examples of maps with leverage fractions less than 1 will be provided.

In the first example (Frances, Map 1), one volunteer staffer (VS) provided a repeated service to one cl-I-ent (C) during the period between March and April, 1997. The results level was ACT3→LEV3. The action points earned by the program (i.e., results level times population multiplier) were 3 × 1 = 3 (note: a population multiplier of 1 and not 0 was used, since the change agent was a volunteer and not a paid staff person). The recipient points earned were also 3 × 1 = 3. The action points were for village building; the recipient points represented cl-I-ent services.

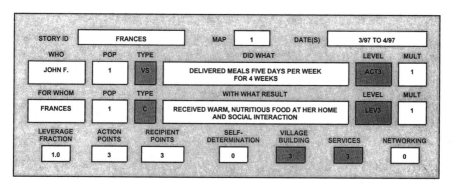

In the next example (Frances, Map 2), the same two parties were interacting. But here, the results level was ACT2→LEV2. Thus, the points earned by the program were 2 × 1 = 2 action points and 2 × 1 = 2 recipient points.

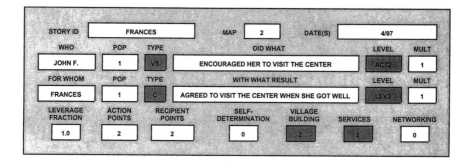

The next example (Frances, Map 3) provides our first case of multiple change agents. Here there were several staff persons involved with the one cl-I-ent. The population of "2" is assigned, by convention, since there were multiple staff involved at various points and viewed as a collective. However, since they were paid staff, the population multiplier applied is "0" (and not "2"). The results level was ACT3→LEV3. Therefore, the program earned 3 × 1 = 3 recipient points, but 3 × 0 = 0 action points. The recipient points were cl-I-ent services.

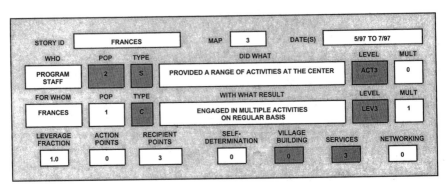

In the next example (Frances, Map 5), the cl-I-ent took action for self-benefit (milestone 4). She was the change agent, there was no separate recipient. The program thus earned 4 × 1 = 4 action points, but no recipient points, for this cl-I-ent action. The 4 points were classified as self-determination.

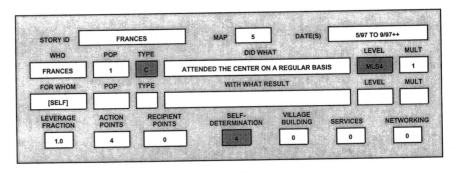

In the next example (Frances, Map 6), the cl-I-ent became a change agent by assisting with meal preparations for the Meals on Wheels program. As such, she was a village builder. However, since she was not in direct contact with the recipients of the meals, the recipient population used was "0" and not the number of persons receiving the meals. Therefore, the program earned 3 × 1= 3 action points, but 3 × 0 = 0 recipient points for her specific efforts here as a village builder.

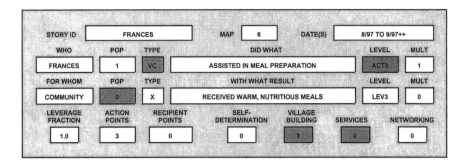

Our next example (PHP-SS, Map 1) provides the first opportunity to see the population multiplier applied. Here, two staff recruited nine community members. The results level was ACT2→LEV2. The population multiplier applied to the change agents was "0," since they were staff (S). A population multiplier of 3 was applied for the nine parents (refer back to Table 6.1). Thus, the program earned 2 × 3 = 6 recipient points, but 2 × 0 = 0 action points. These recipient points were cl-I-ent services.

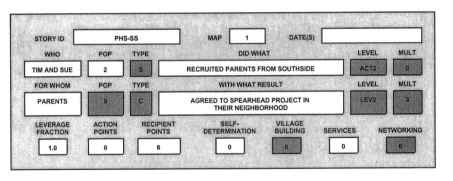

In the next example (PHP-SS, Map 7), a team of six parents attained a team milestone coded as MLS4. Since they were functioning here as a collective (coded as G for group), the population number applied was "2" (which also carried a population multiplier of 2). This resulted in the program earning 4 × 2 = 8 action points. Actions of this type are coded as self-determination points to emphasize the personal growth and self-efficacy of the change agents. No recipient points were earned, since the benefits from their milestone for other community members were in the future. As the center begins operating, additional maps would be added to the story to document the services received.

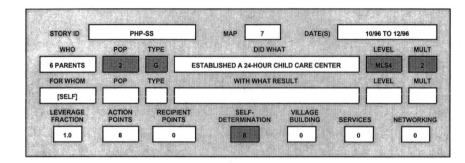

The next example (PHP-SS, Map 11) is also a case in which self-determination points were earned by the program. Here, one cl-I-ent attained MLS4 by returning to school. Again, there are no recipient points earned for this map.

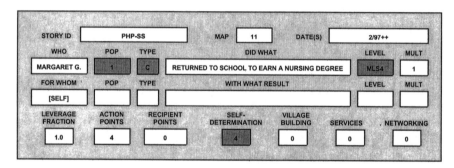

The next example (Jimmy, Maps 2 and 3) illustrates a handoff. In Map 2, a staffer made the referral to the free clinic where volunteer medical and health professionals offer free services to those with needs (coded as G for group). Since this was a handoff, the clinic population, by convention, is "1." For this map, the program earned $2 \times 1 = 2$ recipient points, but $2 \times 0 = 0$ action points. The points were classified as networking. In Map 3, the population assigned to the clinic is "2," by convention. Although the clinic, not the program, provided the service to the cl-I-ent, the program still earned both the $3 \times 2 = 6$ action points (village-building) and the $3 \times 1 = 3$ recipient points (cl-I-ent services)—since full leveraging applied. Note that in Map 3, a "V" is added to the code for the clinic to indicate that the services were provided by volunteers (and thus earned village-building points).

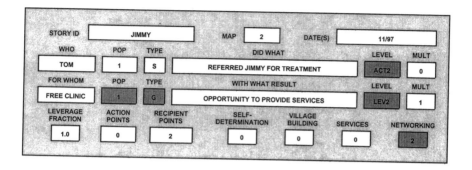

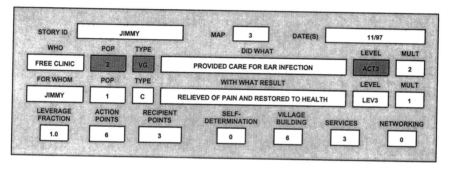

In the next example (Tanya, Map 9), ABC Corp (coded as "G" for organization) offered the program's cl-I-ent a full-time job. The results level was ACT3→LEV3. Although the population assigned to the organization was "2," the multiplier applied was "0," since this change agent was not a volunteer organization. Therefore, the program earned 3 × 1 = 3 recipient points (coded as cl-I-ent services), but no action points (3 × 0 = 0).

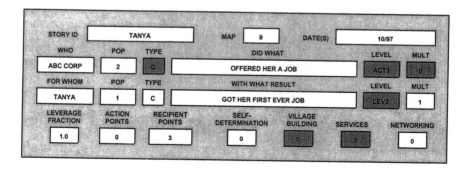

# SPLIT MAPS

For maps in which there are multiple change agents that include both volunteers and paid professionals, we face a dilemma. Should village-building points be earned or not and, if so, how many? To resolve this special case, *split maps* are used. These are multiple maps, each carrying the same Map code but with an "a," "b," or "c" affixed to that number (e.g., Maps 4a and 4b). The recipient information and scoring appears only once, in the map with the "a" code. For the "b" or "c" maps, the For Whom entry is written as "[see above]" and the recipient population is "0." This allows village-building points to be awarded, where appropriate, without double counting of the service points.

To illustrate, in a story including a community picnic, two program staff, a volunteer organization, and seven volunteers from the community worked together to plan and implement the event. Two hundred community members attended the picnic, where they socialized and had opportunities to gain information at booths representing various community services. Their efforts appeared in the story as a split map (Lands End, Maps 5a, 5b, and 5c):

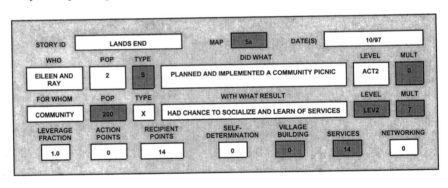

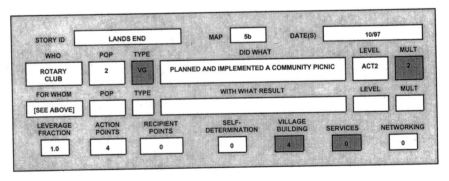

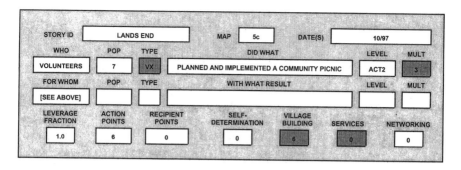

Through the use of the split map, the program earned the 2 × 7 = 14 recipient points for the impact (classified as community services) on the 200 persons attending the picnic, as well as the 2 × 2 = 4 village building points for the work of the volunteer organization and the 2 × 3 = 6 additional village-building points for the efforts of the seven individuals.

# QUIZ 6

6.1. How is progress different on a developmental hierarchy (stage-to-stage development) than on the Results Ladder?

6.2. What is the dilemma facing *staff-driven* programs when it comes to scoring more points based on Results Mapping? What is the way out of this dilemma?

6.3. Why should a program be interested in increasing the percentage of story points earned that are associated with non-staff actions?

6.4. If a program is a short-term service provider, but also networks with other agencies that engage in longer-term interactions with cl-I-ents, can the program ever earn points when one of its cl-I-ents achieves a long-term milestone (i.e., MLS6 or MLS7)?

6.5. Can a program ever earn full credit for a self-referential map coded as MLS7?

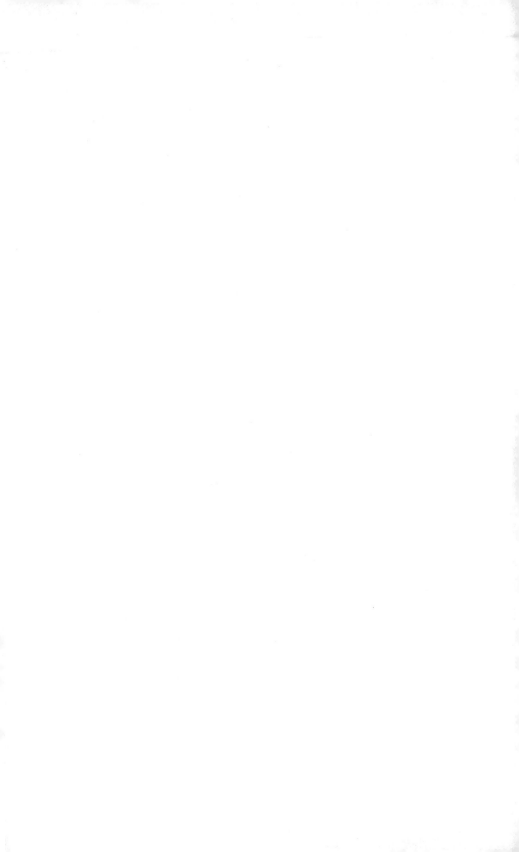

# 7

# Examples of Mapped Stories

I have selected three stories to illustrate the various mapping conventions and scoring rules. As earlier noted, all stories and examples in the book are based on actual cases but have been edited to serve here as training tools while also protecting the confidentiality of clients and programs. The first two stories feature individual program cl-I-ents. The third story focuses on a teen court and involves multiple cl-I-ents.

## STORY 1

Fred is now 15 years of age and a freshman at a local high school in western Montana. Because of academic deficiencies, as well as a series of disciplinary problems last year, he had to repeat the eighth grade. He was very unhappy about this and admitted to plans to make the school year a living hell for other students, teachers, and administrators alike. His case was referred to Bill, the local substance abuse prevention coordinator, when a teacher discovered Fred standing outside the school building smoking a joint. Although funded by the State and not a school employee, Bill maintained a part-time office at the school to be "close to the action."

After some initial tension, Bill and Fred began to communicate. Bill learned that Fred's one joy in life was playing the guitar; but his parents could not afford lessons for him and his old guitar was broken beyond repair. Bill offered Fred a deal: If he was able to secure an acoustic guitar for Fred and arrange for private lessons each lunch hour, would Fred agree to practice each day, behave himself at school during the rest of the day, and attend to his studies? Fred was doubtful that Bill could keep his part of the agreement, but said he would go along.

Bill went to the school principal to present the case. The principal agreed to contribute $350 from her discretional fund and said that she could make a room available during lunch hour for the practice sessions. Bill next went to the local music store, and after much haggling, got the owner to agree to provide a guitar that retailed for $800 for the amount the principal had set aside. Bill brought Fred to the store the next day, after school, and was delighted to see Fred's expression when he was handed the guitar.

Bill found two students in the music department at the local junior college who needed to satisfy a community service requirement. Each agreed to spend two lunch periods a week with Fred for three months. Bill, who had played the guitar a bit in college, assumed responsibility for the remaining day. The lessons began in early October. In January, one of the students—who had taken a liking to Fred— agreed to continue with the lessons through May. Bill, who by then had become Fred's "mentor," in the boy's own words, increased his commitment to three days each week. One afternoon, Fred told Bill that he had stopped using drugs.

By May, Fred was good enough to be invited to be the featured performer in the school graduation ceremony. He had finished the year with no unexcused absences and only one disciplinary action (compared with six such absences and four disciplinary actions the previous year). His lowest grade was a "C" in English, also a major improvement from the previous year.

## Story 1 Mapped

Map 0 is used to provide background for the story. It is not coded or scored.

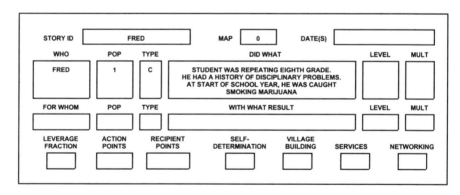

Map 1 highlights the first encounter between the program (represented by Bill) and the cl-I-ent, Fred. Bill took the time to get to know Fred and arrive at a strategy for building on Fred's interests. This was more a service than a simple information transfer and so was coded as ACT3➔LEV3 (rather than at results level 2).

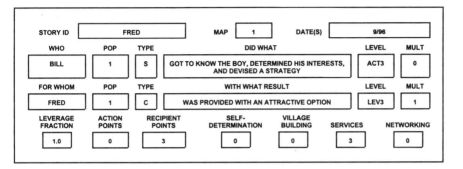

The next two maps (Maps 2 and 3) present Bill's negotiations with the school principal and the music store owner. These can each be interpreted as the first half of a handoff (from Bill to the principal and from Bill to the store owner). The principal was coded as "P" (for provider), since she was doing her job. The music store owner was also coded as "P" (for provider), since he was the only person from the store involved in the transaction. If several persons at the store had been involved, the code would have been "G" (for group) and carried a population of "2"; but this was not the case.

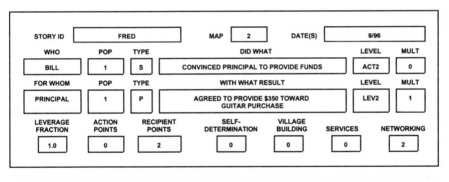

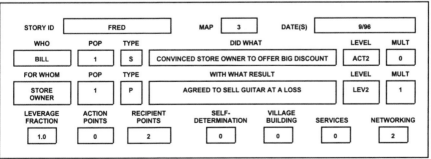

The next three maps (Maps 4a, 4b, 4c) complete the handoffs and result in Fred's obtaining the guitar. This was an "assisted handoff," since Bill was also a key change agent in the transaction. Since both Bill and the principal were doing their jobs, no points were earned for their maps. The maps were included to provide complete documentation of what transpired. In Map 4a, the music owner was considered a village builder (hence the code "VP"), since he provided the guitar at a significantly reduced price (actually at a loss).

| STORY ID | FRED | | MAP | 4a | DATE(S) | 9/96 | |
|---|---|---|---|---|---|---|---|
| WHO | POP | TYPE | DID WHAT | | | LEVEL | MULT |
| STORE OWNER | 1 | VP | SOLD GUITAR AT A LOSS (VOLUNTEER ACT) | | | ACT3 | 1 |
| FOR WHOM | POP | TYPE | WITH WHAT RESULT | | | LEVEL | MULT |
| FRED | 1 | C | RECEIVED AN ACOUSTIC GUITAR | | | LEV3 | 1 |
| LEVERAGE FRACTION | ACTION POINTS | RECIPIENT POINTS | SELF-DETERMINATION | VILLAGE BUILDING | SERVICES | | NETWORKING |
| 1.0 | 3 | 3 | 0 | 3 | 3 | | 0 |

| STORY ID | FRED | | MAP | 4b | DATE(S) | 9/96 | |
|---|---|---|---|---|---|---|---|
| WHO | POP | TYPE | DID WHAT | | | LEVEL | MULT |
| PRINCIPAL | 1 | P | CONTRIBUTED $350 TOWARD PURCHASE OF GUITAR | | | ACT3 | 0 |
| FOR WHOM | POP | TYPE | WITH WHAT RESULT | | | LEVEL | MULT |
| [SEE ABOVE] | | | | | | | |
| LEVERAGE FRACTION | ACTION POINTS | RECIPIENT POINTS | SELF-DETERMINATION | VILLAGE BUILDING | SERVICES | | NETWORKING |
| 1.0 | 0 | 0 | 0 | 0 | 0 | | 0 |

| STORY ID | FRED | | MAP | 4c | DATE(S) | 9/96 | |
|---|---|---|---|---|---|---|---|
| WHO | POP | TYPE | DID WHAT | | | LEVEL | MULT |
| BILL | 1 | S | TOOK FRED TO STORE TO OBTAIN GUITAR | | | ACT2 | 0 |
| FOR WHOM | POP | TYPE | WITH WHAT RESULT | | | LEVEL | MULT |
| [SEE ABOVE] | | | | | | | |
| LEVERAGE FRACTION | ACTION POINTS | RECIPIENT POINTS | SELF-DETERMINATION | VILLAGE BUILDING | SERVICES | | NETWORKING |
| 1.0 | 0 | 0 | 0 | 0 | 0 | | 0 |

The next map (Map 5) deals with the recruitment of the two junior college students. Since they will be providing services as community service, they will be coded as "VX" (volunteers from the community) and earn village building points for their actions as change agents in subsequent maps. Recruitment, by convention, is coded as ACT2→LEV2.

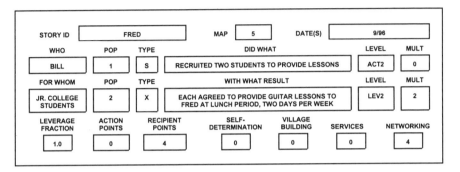

The next set of maps (Maps 6–12) covers the guitar lessons. For the first junior college student, there was a single map (Map 6), since his role as change agent lasted only three months. For the second student, there were three maps (Maps 7–9) since he was active for eight months (one map for each three months of repeated service). Their interaction with Fred was ACT3→LEV3. Bill's situation was different. In addition to providing lessons, he developed a mentoring relationship with Fred (coded as ACT5→LEV5). However, since it takes six months—by convention—to map a mentoring relationship at Level 5, the first two maps showing the interactions between Bill and Fred (Maps 10 and 11) were coded as ACT3→LEV3.

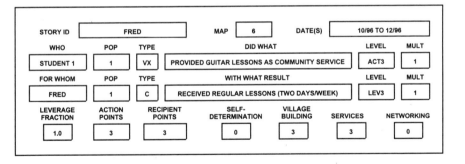

| STORY ID | FRED | | MAP | 7 | DATE(S) | 10/96 TO 12/96 |

| WHO | POP | TYPE | DID WHAT | LEVEL | MULT |
|---|---|---|---|---|---|
| STUDENT 2 | 1 | VX | PROVIDED GUITAR LESSONS AS COMMUNITY SERVICE | ACT3 | 1 |

| FOR WHOM | POP | TYPE | WITH WHAT RESULT | LEVEL | MULT |
|---|---|---|---|---|---|
| FRED | 1 | C | RECEIVED REGULAR LESSONS (TWO DAYS/WEEK) | LEV3 | 1 |

| LEVERAGE FRACTION | ACTION POINTS | RECIPIENT POINTS | SELF-DETERMINATION | VILLAGE BUILDING | SERVICES | NETWORKING |
|---|---|---|---|---|---|---|
| 1.0 | 3 | 3 | 0 | 3 | 3 | 0 |

---

| STORY ID | FRED | | MAP | 8 | DATE(S) | 1/97 TO 3/97 |

| WHO | POP | TYPE | DID WHAT | LEVEL | MULT |
|---|---|---|---|---|---|
| STUDENT 2 | 1 | VX | PROVIDED GUITAR LESSONS AS COMMUNITY SERVICE | ACT3 | 1 |

| FOR WHOM | POP | TYPE | WITH WHAT RESULT | LEVEL | MULT |
|---|---|---|---|---|---|
| FRED | 1 | C | RECEIVED REGULAR LESSONS (TWO DAYS/WEEK) | LEV3 | 1 |

| LEVERAGE FRACTION | ACTION POINTS | RECIPIENT POINTS | SELF-DETERMINATION | VILLAGE BUILDING | SERVICES | NETWORKING |
|---|---|---|---|---|---|---|
| 1.0 | 3 | 3 | 0 | 3 | 3 | 0 |

---

| STORY ID | FRED | | MAP | 9 | DATE(S) | 4/97 TO 5/97 |

| WHO | POP | TYPE | DID WHAT | LEVEL | MULT |
|---|---|---|---|---|---|
| STUDENT 2 | 1 | VX | PROVIDED GUITAR LESSONS AS COMMUNITY SERVICE | ACT3 | 1 |

| FOR WHOM | POP | TYPE | WITH WHAT RESULT | LEVEL | MULT |
|---|---|---|---|---|---|
| FRED | 1 | C | RECEIVED REGULAR LESSONS (TWO DAYS/WEEK) | LEV3 | 1 |

| LEVERAGE FRACTION | ACTION POINTS | RECIPIENT POINTS | SELF-DETERMINATION | VILLAGE BUILDING | SERVICES | NETWORKING |
|---|---|---|---|---|---|---|
| 1.0 | 3 | 3 | 0 | 3 | 3 | 0 |

---

| STORY ID | FRED | | MAP | 10 | DATE(S) | 10/96 TO 12/96 |

| WHO | POP | TYPE | DID WHAT | LEVEL | MULT |
|---|---|---|---|---|---|
| BILL | 1 | S | PROVIDED GUITAR LESSONS AND MENTORED | ACT3 | 0 |

| FOR WHOM | POP | TYPE | WITH WHAT RESULT | LEVEL | MULT |
|---|---|---|---|---|---|
| FRED | 1 | C | RECEIVED REGULAR LESSONS (ONE DAY/WEEK) AND SUPPORT FROM A CARING ADULT | LEV3 | 1 |

| LEVERAGE FRACTION | ACTION POINTS | RECIPIENT POINTS | SELF-DETERMINATION | VILLAGE BUILDING | SERVICES | NETWORKING |
|---|---|---|---|---|---|---|
| 1.0 | 0 | 3 | 0 | 0 | 3 | 0 |

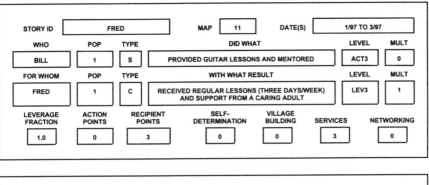

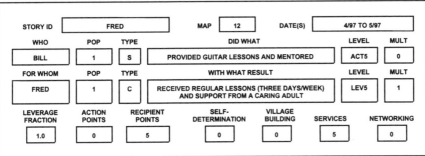

Before going to the end of the story (May–June 1997), were there any milestones to capture thus far? Fred's willingness to attend school regularly, avoid getting into trouble, and practice each lunch hour certainly represented a breakthrough for him. This was coded as a MLS4 after more than one month of this new behavior had elapsed. In addition, he stopped using drugs. This was another clear signal of growth. Again, this deserved a MLS4. These two milestones were mapped next (Maps 13 and 14). Had there not been a MLS4, the relationship between Bill and Fred would have remained and been coded at Level 3 in Map 12 rather than at Level 5.

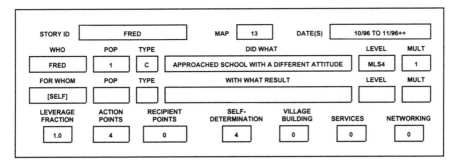

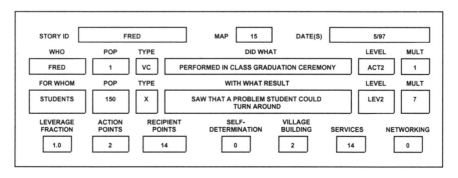

| STORY ID | FRED | MAP | 14 | DATE(S) | 11/96 TO 1/97++ | | | |
|---|---|---|---|---|---|---|---|---|
| WHO | POP | TYPE | DID WHAT | | | LEVEL | MULT | |
| FRED | 1 | C | STOPPED USING DRUGS (AS SELF-REPORTED) | | | MLS4 | 1 | |
| FOR WHOM | POP | TYPE | WITH WHAT RESULT | | | LEVEL | MULT | |
| [SELF] | | | | | | | | |
| LEVERAGE FRACTION | ACTION POINTS | RECIPIENT POINTS | SELF-DETERMINATION | VILLAGE BUILDING | SERVICES | NETWORKING | | |
| 1.0 | 4 | 0 | 4 | 0 | 0 | 0 | | |

In late May, Fred was invited to be the feature performer at his class graduation. As far as anyone could tell, this was the first positive, public recognition ever given to him. In a sense, he had become a "role model" for other students in the school who did not excel in academics or sports. More than 150 students attended the graduation and applauded Fred's performance. This was coded as ACT2→LEV2, with the 150+ students as the recipients and Fred as a "village builder" (Map 15).

| STORY ID | FRED | MAP | 15 | DATE(S) | 5/97 | | | |
|---|---|---|---|---|---|---|---|---|
| WHO | POP | TYPE | DID WHAT | | | LEVEL | MULT | |
| FRED | 1 | VC | PERFORMED IN CLASS GRADUATION CEREMONY | | | ACT2 | 1 | |
| FOR WHOM | POP | TYPE | WITH WHAT RESULT | | | LEVEL | MULT | |
| STUDENTS | 150 | X | SAW THAT A PROBLEM STUDENT COULD TURN AROUND | | | LEV2 | 7 | |
| LEVERAGE FRACTION | ACTION POINTS | RECIPIENT POINTS | SELF-DETERMINATION | VILLAGE BUILDING | SERVICES | NETWORKING | | |
| 1.0 | 2 | 14 | 0 | 2 | 14 | 0 | | |

As final maps of the story (Maps 16 and 17), Fred's longer-term accomplishments are noted. He completed the year with only one disciplinary action (compared with four the previous year) and no unexcused absences (compared with six in the previous school year). His grades were improved. He was heading for high school with decent prospects of not dropping out (as had his two older brothers). These collective achievements are coded as MLS6 in Map 16; and because Bill provided services at results level 5 to help make these achievements possible, the prevention program staffed by Bill earned full credit for this achievement (i.e., the map leverage fraction was 1.0). In addition, Fred still was not using drugs. This was likewise coded as MLS6 and full credit was earned by the program.

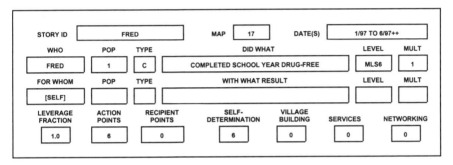

*Story Summary.* Fred's story earned the program 37 action points and 51 recipient points. Of the action points, 20 points represented acts of cl-I-ent self-determination and 17 points represented village building (by the store owner, the two junior college students, and by the cl-I-ent when he performed for his school). Of the recipient points, 29 points were for direct cl-I-ent services, 8 points were for networking (from Bill to the principal, store owner, and junior college students), and the remaining 14 points reflected the "motivational impact" on Fred's peers. The program staffer (i.e., Bill) was the change agent in exactly half of the 16 maps, with most of his activity at results level 3 (interacting with Fred)—but ultimately growing into a results level 5 relationship with the cl-I-ent. Fred achieved four milestones, two at MLS4 and two at MLS6.

# STORY 2

Rick was diagnosed with HIV in 1990 and was later diagnosed with AIDS in 1994. Throughout that period, he had a history of urinary infections, dizziness, weakness and fatigue, difficulties with activities of daily living, lack of concentration, and memory problems. By late 1994, Rick was in and out of the hospital and his overall living situation was not stable. He was living with two roommates and was having problems with the landlord, finances, and his health.

Rick was referred to the program's AIDS project on September 9, 1994. Initially, a staff member assisted Rick in gaining access to all state and Federal benefits to which he was entitled. Since he was in and out of the hospital, a second staff member was involved with him and his mother, Jane, in discharge planning and obtaining durable medical equipment for his apartment. By late April 1995, Rick's mental and physical health deteriorated sharply. The staffer provided continual support to Rick and especially to his mother. Due to poor health and ongoing housing issues, Rick moved in with Jane in June so that Jane could tend to his needs more readily.

From May 1995 through February 1996, Rick was not getting any better and the staffer referred issues regarding creditors/debts to AIDS Legal Services. She also worked with a funeral home to obtain information regarding pre-planned funeral services for the family, with ARIS to provide respite services to Jane, and with Outreach to provide paratransit transportation services for Rick. Throughout this time, a third staffer was working with the state to insure that benefits for Rick would remain intact. The second staffer served as the case manager and was viewed by both Rick and Jane as a continual source of hope, support, and strength.

Miraculously, after April 1996, Rick became more alert and oriented. His health improved greatly (his CD4 count rose and his viral load count was down). He began assuming a normal lifestyle. Since July, he has served as a motivational speaker through the Speaker Bureau and has talked with over 600 AIDS victims and their families regarding his experiences with HIV/AIDS.

The program provided this story in September 1997 for inclusion in an annual evaluation report sponsored by one of its funders, The Health Trust in Campbell, California. The program's initial involvement with the cl-I-ent and his mother dated back to the 1994–95 period. Following our convention, only maps dated after September 1995 were scored (i.e., points earned within two years of the evaluation cut-off date). Earlier maps were presented to provide background for the maps that were scored and included in the evaluation.

# Story 2 Mapped

Map 0 summarized Rick's case.

| STORY ID | RICK | | MAP | 0 | DATE(S) | |
|---|---|---|---|---|---|---|

| WHO | POP | TYPE | DID WHAT | LEVEL | MULT |
|---|---|---|---|---|---|
| RICK | 1 | C | HE WAS DIAGNOSED WITH AIDS IN 1994. BY LATE 1994, HE WAS IN AND OUT OF THE HOSPITAL AND HIS OVERALL LIVING SITUATION WAS NOT STABLE. | | |

| FOR WHOM | POP | TYPE | WITH WHAT RESULT | LEVEL | MULT |
|---|---|---|---|---|---|
| | | | | | |

| LEVERAGE FRACTION | ACTION POINTS | RECIPIENT POINTS | SELF-DETERMINATION | VILLAGE BUILDING | SERVICES | NETWORKING |
|---|---|---|---|---|---|---|
| 1.0 | | | | | | |

Maps 1 through 4 present the initial services provided to Rick and to Jane, his mother, who—after June 1995—became his primary care giver. As noted, these early maps were not coded (with results levels) or scored. For this reason, Maps 3 and 4, which span many months, were not broken up into three-month segments.

| STORY ID | RICK | | MAP | 1 | DATE(S) | 9/94 |
|---|---|---|---|---|---|---|

| WHO | POP | TYPE | DID WHAT | LEVEL | MULT |
|---|---|---|---|---|---|
| STAFFER #1 | 1 | S | PROVIDED BENEFIT COUNSELING SERVICES | | |

| FOR WHOM | POP | TYPE | WITH WHAT RESULT | LEVEL | MULT |
|---|---|---|---|---|---|
| RICK | 1 | C | GAINED ACCESS TO ALL STATE AND FEDERAL BENEFITS TO WHICH HE WAS ENTITLED | | |

| LEVERAGE FRACTION | ACTION POINTS | RECIPIENT POINTS | SELF-DETERMINATION | VILLAGE BUILDING | SERVICES | NETWORKING |
|---|---|---|---|---|---|---|
| 1.0 | | | | | | |

| STORY ID | RICK | | MAP | 2 | DATE(S) | 11/94 TO 12/94 |
|---|---|---|---|---|---|---|

| WHO | POP | TYPE | DID WHAT | LEVEL | MULT |
|---|---|---|---|---|---|
| STAFFER #2 | 1 | S | ASSISTED WITH HOSPITAL DISCHARGE AND OBTAINED GRAB BARS AND BATH BENCH FOR APARTMENT | | |

| FOR WHOM | POP | TYPE | WITH WHAT RESULT | LEVEL | MULT |
|---|---|---|---|---|---|
| RICK | 1 | C | PROVIDED WITH A SAFE HOME ENVIRONMENT | | |

| LEVERAGE FRACTION | ACTION POINTS | RECIPIENT POINTS | SELF-DETERMINATION | VILLAGE BUILDING | SERVICES | NETWORKING |
|---|---|---|---|---|---|---|
| 1.0 | | | | | | |

| STORY ID | RICK | | | MAP | 3 | DATE(S) | 4/95 TO 8/96 |
|---|---|---|---|---|---|---|---|

| WHO | POP | TYPE | DID WHAT | LEVEL | MULT |
|---|---|---|---|---|---|
| STAFFER #2 | 1 | S | PROVIDED ON-GOING COUNSELING AND SUPPORT | | |

| FOR WHOM | POP | TYPE | WITH WHAT RESULT | LEVEL | MULT |
|---|---|---|---|---|---|
| RICK | 1 | C | DECREASED STRESS AND ANXIETY | | |

| LEVERAGE FRACTION | ACTION POINTS | RECIPIENT POINTS | SELF-DETERMINATION | VILLAGE BUILDING | SERVICES | NETWORKING |
|---|---|---|---|---|---|---|
| 1.0 | | | | | | |

---

| STORY ID | RICK | | | MAP | 4 | DATE(S) | 4/95 TO 8/96 |
|---|---|---|---|---|---|---|---|

| WHO | POP | TYPE | DID WHAT | LEVEL | MULT |
|---|---|---|---|---|---|
| STAFFER #2 | 1 | S | PROVIDED ON-GOING COUNSELING AND SUPPORT | | |

| FOR WHOM | POP | TYPE | WITH WHAT RESULT | LEVEL | MULT |
|---|---|---|---|---|---|
| JANE | 1 | F | DECREASED STRESS AND ANXIETY AND ABLE TO ASSUME GREATER RESPONSIBILITY AS CARE GIVER | | |

| LEVERAGE FRACTION | ACTION POINTS | RECIPIENT POINTS | SELF-DETERMINATION | VILLAGE BUILDING | SERVICES | NETWORKING |
|---|---|---|---|---|---|---|
| 1.0 | | | | | | |

The next ten maps (Maps 5 through 14) involved four handoffs by the program to other local service providers. In each case, the first map in the pair showed the handoff while the second map (and third map in two cases where services were provided for longer than three months) indicated the services provided to either Rick or Jane. By convention, the handoff was coded as ACT2→LEV2. The follow-through services provided were coded as ACT3→LEV3, with the exception of those provided by the funeral home (Map 8), which were limited to information and therefore coded as results level 2. While Rick received many of these services at no cost, the service providers were reimbursed for their time and expenses through various grants and public funds. Therefore, there was no village building associated with these activities. The programs were coded as "G" (for group) and assigned population values of "1," by convention, when they received handoffs and "2" when they delivered services.

| STORY ID | RICK | | | MAP | 5 | DATE(S) | 9/95 |
|---|---|---|---|---|---|---|---|

| WHO | POP | TYPE | DID WHAT | LEVEL | MULT |
|---|---|---|---|---|---|
| STAFFER #2 | 1 | S | MADE REFERRAL | ACT2 | 0 |

| FOR WHOM | POP | TYPE | WITH WHAT RESULT | LEVEL | MULT |
|---|---|---|---|---|---|
| AIDS LEGAL SERVICES | 1 | G | ENABLED TO ASSIST CLIENT WITH ISSUES REGARDING CREDITORS AND DEBTS | LEV2 | 1 |

| LEVERAGE FRACTION | ACTION POINTS | RECIPIENT POINTS | SELF-DETERMINATION | VILLAGE BUILDING | SERVICES | NETWORKING |
|---|---|---|---|---|---|---|
| 1.0 | 0 | 2 | 0 | 0 | 0 | 2 |

| STORY ID | RICK | | MAP | 6 | DATE(S) | 9/95 | |
|---|---|---|---|---|---|---|---|
| WHO | POP | TYPE | DID WHAT | | | LEVEL | MULT |
| AIDS LEGAL SERVICES | 2 | G | ASSISTED IN LETTER WRITING AND DIRECT CONTACTS WITH CREDITORS | | | ACT3 | 0 |
| FOR WHOM | POP | TYPE | WITH WHAT RESULT | | | LEVEL | MULT |
| RICK | 1 | C | RESOLVED HIS CREDITOR ISSUES | | | LEV3 | 1 |

| LEVERAGE FRACTION | ACTION POINTS | RECIPIENT POINTS | SELF-DETERMINATION | VILLAGE BUILDING | SERVICES | NETWORKING |
|---|---|---|---|---|---|---|
| 1.0 | 0 | 3 | 0 | 0 | 3 | 0 |

| STORY ID | RICK | | MAP | 7 | DATE(S) | 10/95 | |
|---|---|---|---|---|---|---|---|
| WHO | POP | TYPE | DID WHAT | | | LEVEL | MULT |
| STAFFER #2 | 1 | S | ARRANGED MEETING | | | ACT2 | 0 |
| FOR WHOM | POP | TYPE | WITH WHAT RESULT | | | LEVEL | MULT |
| FUNERAL HOME | 1 | G | ENABLED TO ASSIST FAMILY BY DISCUSSING PRE-PLANNING SERVICES | | | LEV2 | 1 |

| LEVERAGE FRACTION | ACTION POINTS | RECIPIENT POINTS | SELF-DETERMINATION | VILLAGE BUILDING | SERVICES | NETWORKING |
|---|---|---|---|---|---|---|
| 1.0 | 0 | 2 | 0 | 0 | 0 | 2 |

| STORY ID | RICK | | MAP | 8 | DATE(S) | 10/95 | |
|---|---|---|---|---|---|---|---|
| WHO | POP | TYPE | DID WHAT | | | LEVEL | MULT |
| FUNERAL HOME | 2 | G | PROVIDED INFORMATION ON PRE-PLANNING FUNERAL SERVICES | | | ACT2 | 0 |
| FOR WHOM | POP | TYPE | WITH WHAT RESULT | | | LEVEL | MULT |
| JANE | 1 | F | LEARNED OF OPTIONS AND COSTS | | | LEV2 | 1 |

| LEVERAGE FRACTION | ACTION POINTS | RECIPIENT POINTS | SELF-DETERMINATION | VILLAGE BUILDING | SERVICES | NETWORKING |
|---|---|---|---|---|---|---|
| 1.0 | 0 | 2 | 0 | 0 | 2 | 0 |

| STORY ID | RICK | | MAP | 9 | DATE(S) | 11/95 | |
|---|---|---|---|---|---|---|---|
| WHO | POP | TYPE | DID WHAT | | | LEVEL | MULT |
| STAFFER #2 | 1 | S | REFERRED CASE TO RESPITE GROUP | | | ACT2 | 0 |
| FOR WHOM | POP | TYPE | WITH WHAT RESULT | | | LEVEL | MULT |
| ARIS | 1 | G | ENABLED TO ASSIST PRIMARY CARE GIVER | | | LEV2 | 1 |

| LEVERAGE FRACTION | ACTION POINTS | RECIPIENT POINTS | SELF-DETERMINATION | VILLAGE BUILDING | SERVICES | NETWORKING |
|---|---|---|---|---|---|---|
| 1.0 | 0 | 2 | 0 | 0 | 0 | 2 |

| STORY ID | | RICK | MAP | 10 | DATE(S) | | 11/95 TO 1/96 |
|---|---|---|---|---|---|---|---|

| WHO | POP | TYPE | DID WHAT | | | LEVEL | MULT |
|---|---|---|---|---|---|---|---|
| ARIS | 2 | G | PROVIDED A CARE GIVER FOR RESPITE SUPPORT | | | ACT3 | 0 |

| FOR WHOM | POP | TYPE | WITH WHAT RESULT | | | LEVEL | MULT |
|---|---|---|---|---|---|---|---|
| JANE | 1 | F | ABLE TO MAINTAIN MENTAL HEALTH UNDER STRESSFUL LIFE SITUATION | | | LEV3 | 1 |

| LEVERAGE FRACTION | ACTION POINTS | RECIPIENT POINTS | SELF-DETERMINATION | VILLAGE BUILDING | SERVICES | NETWORKING |
|---|---|---|---|---|---|---|
| 1.0 | 0 | 3 | 0 | 0 | 3 | 0 |

---

| STORY ID | | RICK | MAP | 11 | DATE(S) | | 2/96 TO 3/96 |
|---|---|---|---|---|---|---|---|

| WHO | POP | TYPE | DID WHAT | | | LEVEL | MULT |
|---|---|---|---|---|---|---|---|
| ARIS | 2 | | A CARE GIVER FOR RESPITE SUPPORT | | | ACT3 | 0 |

| FOR WHOM | POP | TYPE | WITH WHAT RESULT | | | LEVEL | MULT |
|---|---|---|---|---|---|---|---|
| JANE | 1 | F | ABLE TO MAINTAIN MENTAL HEALTH UNDER STRESSFUL LIFE SITUATION | | | LEV3 | 1 |

| LEVERAGE FRACTION | ACTION POINTS | RECIPIENT POINTS | SELF-DETERMINATION | VILLAGE BUILDING | SERVICES | NETWORKING |
|---|---|---|---|---|---|---|
| 1.0 | 0 | 3 | 0 | 0 | 3 | 0 |

---

| STORY ID | | RICK | MAP | 12 | DATE(S) | | 11/95 |
|---|---|---|---|---|---|---|---|

| WHO | POP | TYPE | DID WHAT | | | LEVEL | MULT |
|---|---|---|---|---|---|---|---|
| STAFFER #2 | 1 | S | ASSISTED WITH APPLICATION AND REFERRAL | | | ACT2 | 0 |

| FOR WHOM | POP | TYPE | WITH WHAT RESULT | | | LEVEL | MULT |
|---|---|---|---|---|---|---|---|
| OUTREACH INC. | 1 | G | ENABLED TO ASSIST CLIENT | | | LEV2 | 1 |

| LEVERAGE FRACTION | ACTION POINTS | RECIPIENT POINTS | SELF-DETERMINATION | VILLAGE BUILDING | SERVICES | NETWORKING |
|---|---|---|---|---|---|---|
| 1.0 | 0 | 2 | 0 | 0 | 0 | 2 |

---

| STORY ID | | RICK | MAP | 13 | DATE(S) | | 11/95 TO 1/96 |
|---|---|---|---|---|---|---|---|

| WHO | POP | TYPE | DID WHAT | | | LEVEL | MULT |
|---|---|---|---|---|---|---|---|
| OUTREACH INC. | 2 | G | PROVIDED PARATRANSIT TRANSPORTATION SERVICES | | | ACT3 | 0 |

| FOR WHOM | POP | TYPE | WITH WHAT RESULT | | | LEVEL | MULT |
|---|---|---|---|---|---|---|---|
| RICK | 1 | C | ABLE TO GET TO APPOINTMENTS AND VISIT FRIENDS | | | LEV3 | 1 |

| LEVERAGE FRACTION | ACTION POINTS | RECIPIENT POINTS | SELF-DETERMINATION | VILLAGE BUILDING | SERVICES | NETWORKING |
|---|---|---|---|---|---|---|
| 1.0 | 0 | 3 | 0 | 0 | 3 | 0 |

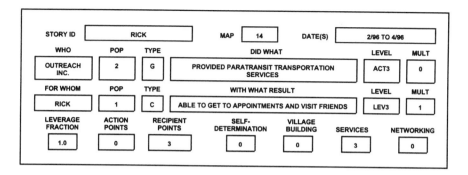

The next nine maps (Maps 15–20b) show ongoing work of the program staff in providing direct services to Rick and Jane. Note that the relationship developed with staffer #2 had already evolved to ACT5→LEV5 by September 1995 when the scoring of the story began. The six maps showing this relationship (Maps 18a–20b) were split so that cl-I-ent services could be distinguished from family member services (for subsequent analysis).

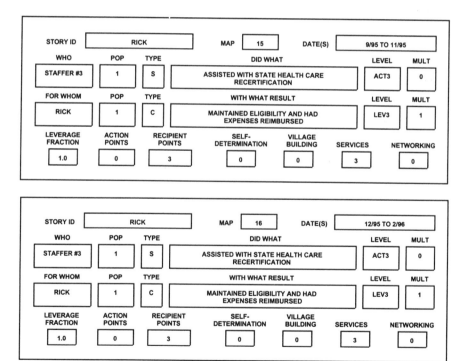

| STORY ID | RICK | | MAP | 17 | DATE(S) | 3/96 TO 4/96 |
|----------|------|--|-----|-----|---------|--------------|

| WHO | POP | TYPE | DID WHAT | LEVEL | MULT |
|-----|-----|------|----------|-------|------|
| STAFFER #3 | 1 | S | ASSISTED WITH STATE HEALTH CARE RECERTIFICATION | ACT3 | 0 |

| FOR WHOM | POP | TYPE | WITH WHAT RESULT | LEVEL | MULT |
|----------|-----|------|------------------|-------|------|
| RICK | 1 | C | MAINTAINED ELIGIBILITY AND HAD EXPENSES REIMBURSED | LEV3 | 1 |

| LEVERAGE FRACTION | ACTION POINTS | RECIPIENT POINTS | SELF-DETERMINATION | VILLAGE BUILDING | SERVICES | NETWORKING |
|-------------------|---------------|------------------|--------------------|------------------|----------|------------|
| 1.0 | 0 | 3 | 0 | 0 | 3 | 0 |

---

| STORY ID | RICK | | MAP | 18a | DATE(S) | 9/95 TO 11/95 |
|----------|------|--|-----|-----|---------|---------------|

| WHO | POP | TYPE | DID WHAT | LEVEL | MULT |
|-----|-----|------|----------|-------|------|
| STAFFER #2 | 1 | S | PROVIDED ON-GOING SUPPORT, STRENGTH, HOPE | ACT5 | 0 |

| FOR WHOM | POP | TYPE | WITH WHAT RESULT | LEVEL | MULT |
|----------|-----|------|------------------|-------|------|
| RICK | 1 | C | RELIEVED OF STRESS (ENABLED TO HEAL) | LEV5 | 1 |

| LEVERAGE FRACTION | ACTION POINTS | RECIPIENT POINTS | SELF-DETERMINATION | VILLAGE BUILDING | SERVICES | NETWORKING |
|-------------------|---------------|------------------|--------------------|------------------|----------|------------|
| 1.0 | 0 | 5 | 0 | 0 | 5 | 0 |

---

| STORY ID | RICK | | MAP | 18b | DATE(S) | 8/95 TO 11/95 |
|----------|------|--|-----|-----|---------|---------------|

| WHO | POP | TYPE | DID WHAT | LEVEL | MULT |
|-----|-----|------|----------|-------|------|
| STAFFER #2 | 1 | S | [SEE ABOVE] | | |

| FOR WHOM | POP | TYPE | WITH WHAT RESULT | LEVEL | MULT |
|----------|-----|------|------------------|-------|------|
| JANE | 1 | F | RELIEVED OF STRESS (ENABLED TO PROVIDE CARE) | LEV5 | 1 |

| LEVERAGE FRACTION | ACTION POINTS | RECIPIENT POINTS | SELF-DETERMINATION | VILLAGE BUILDING | SERVICES | NETWORKING |
|-------------------|---------------|------------------|--------------------|------------------|----------|------------|
| 1.0 | 0 | 5 | 0 | 0 | 5 | 0 |

---

| STORY ID | RICK | | MAP | 19a | DATE(S) | 12/95 TO 2/96 |
|----------|------|--|-----|-----|---------|---------------|

| WHO | POP | TYPE | DID WHAT | LEVEL | MULT |
|-----|-----|------|----------|-------|------|
| STAFFER #2 | 1 | S | PROVIDED ON-GOING SUPPORT, STRENGTH, HOPE | ACT5 | 0 |

| FOR WHOM | POP | TYPE | WITH WHAT RESULT | LEVEL | MULT |
|----------|-----|------|------------------|-------|------|
| RICK | 1 | C | RELIEVED OF STRESS (ENABLED TO HEAL) | LEV5 | 1 |

| LEVERAGE FRACTION | ACTION POINTS | RECIPIENT POINTS | SELF-DETERMINATION | VILLAGE BUILDING | SERVICES | NETWORKING |
|-------------------|---------------|------------------|--------------------|------------------|----------|------------|
| 1.0 | 0 | 5 | 0 | 0 | 5 | 0 |

| STORY ID | RICK | | MAP | 19b | DATE(S) | 12/95 TO 2/96 |
|---|---|---|---|---|---|---|
| WHO | POP | TYPE | DID WHAT | | LEVEL | MULT |
| STAFFER #2 | 1 | S | [SEE ABOVE] | | | |
| FOR WHOM | POP | TYPE | WITH WHAT RESULT | | LEVEL | MULT |
| JANE | 1 | F | RELIEVED OF STRESS (ENABLED TO PROVIDE CARE) | | LEV5 | 1 |

| LEVERAGE FRACTION | ACTION POINTS | RECIPIENT POINTS | SELF-DETERMINATION | VILLAGE BUILDING | SERVICES | NETWORKING |
|---|---|---|---|---|---|---|
| 1.0 | 0 | 5 | 0 | 0 | 5 | 0 |

| STORY ID | RICK | | MAP | 20a | DATE(S) | 3/96 TO 5/96 |
|---|---|---|---|---|---|---|
| WHO | POP | TYPE | DID WHAT | | LEVEL | MULT |
| STAFFER #2 | 1 | S | PROVIDED ON-GOING SUPPORT, STRENGTH, HOPE | | ACT5 | 0 |
| FOR WHOM | POP | TYPE | WITH WHAT RESULT | | LEVEL | MULT |
| RICK | 1 | C | RELIEVED OF STRESS (ENABLED TO HEAL) | | LEV5 | 1 |

| LEVERAGE FRACTION | ACTION POINTS | RECIPIENT POINTS | SELF-DETERMINATION | VILLAGE BUILDING | SERVICES | NETWORKING |
|---|---|---|---|---|---|---|
| 1.0 | 0 | 5 | 0 | 0 | 5 | 0 |

| STORY ID | RICK | | MAP | 20b | DATE(S) | 3/96 TO 5/96 |
|---|---|---|---|---|---|---|
| WHO | POP | TYPE | DID WHAT | | LEVEL | MULT |
| STAFFER #2 | 1 | S | [SEE ABOVE] | | | |
| FOR WHOM | POP | TYPE | WITH WHAT RESULT | | LEVEL | MULT |
| JANE | 1 | F | RELIEVED OF STRESS (ENABLED TO PROVIDE CARE) | | LEV5 | 1 |

| LEVERAGE FRACTION | ACTION POINTS | RECIPIENT POINTS | SELF-DETERMINATION | VILLAGE BUILDING | SERVICES | NETWORKING |
|---|---|---|---|---|---|---|
| 1.0 | 0 | 5 | 0 | 0 | 5 | 0 |

Throughout this period, Jane was the primary care giver to Rick. The support provided by the program, as earlier noted and mapped, allowed her to maintain an ACT5→LEV5 healing relationship with her son. This is shown in Maps 21 through 23 with Jane's efforts categorized as village building.

| STORY ID | RICK | | | MAP | 21 | DATE(S) | 9/95 TO 11/95 | |
|---|---|---|---|---|---|---|---|---|
| WHO | POP | TYPE | DID WHAT | | | | LEVEL | MULT |
| JANE | 1 | VF | PROVIDED ON-GOING SUPPORT, LOVE, AND CARE | | | | ACT5 | 1 |
| FOR WHOM | POP | TYPE | WITH WHAT RESULT | | | | LEVEL | MULT |
| RICK | 1 | C | SUPPORTED IN HEALING PROCESS | | | | LEV5 | 1 |
| LEVERAGE FRACTION | ACTION POINTS | RECIPIENT POINTS | SELF-DETERMINATION | VILLAGE BUILDING | SERVICES | | NETWORKING | |
| 1.0 | 5 | 5 | 0 | 5 | 5 | | 0 | |

| STORY ID | RICK | | | MAP | 22 | DATE(S) | 12/95 TO 2/96 | |
|---|---|---|---|---|---|---|---|---|
| WHO | POP | TYPE | DID WHAT | | | | LEVEL | MULT |
| JANE | 1 | VF | PROVIDED ON-GOING SUPPORT, LOVE, AND CARE | | | | ACT5 | 1 |
| FOR WHOM | POP | TYPE | WITH WHAT RESULT | | | | LEVEL | MULT |
| RICK | 1 | C | SUPPORTED IN HEALING PROCESS | | | | LEV5 | 1 |
| LEVERAGE FRACTION | ACTION POINTS | RECIPIENT POINTS | SELF-DETERMINATION | VILLAGE BUILDING | SERVICES | | NETWORKING | |
| 1.0 | 5 | 5 | 0 | 5 | 5 | | 0 | |

| STORY ID | RICK | | | MAP | 23 | DATE(S) | 3/96 TO 5/96 | |
|---|---|---|---|---|---|---|---|---|
| WHO | POP | TYPE | DID WHAT | | | | LEVEL | MULT |
| JANE | 1 | VF | PROVIDED ON-GOING SUPPORT, LOVE, AND CARE | | | | ACT5 | 1 |
| FOR WHOM | POP | TYPE | WITH WHAT RESULT | | | | LEVEL | MULT |
| RICK | 1 | C | SUPPORTED IN HEALING PROCESS | | | | LEV5 | 1 |
| LEVERAGE FRACTION | ACTION POINTS | RECIPIENT POINTS | SELF-DETERMINATION | VILLAGE BUILDING | SERVICES | | NETWORKING | |
| 1.0 | 5 | 5 | 0 | 5 | 5 | | 0 | |

In the next set of maps (Maps 24–26), the story's milestones are captured. The program rightly claimed that both Rick and his mother reached MLS4 as they came to terms with his illness and needs and took responsible actions. And Rick's recovery process certainly warranted a MLS6. Since a program staffer was involved with the case at results level 5, full credit was given the program for this longer-term milestone.

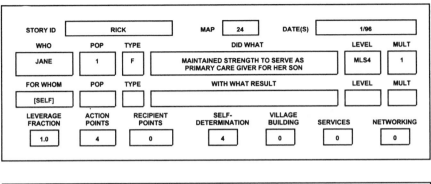

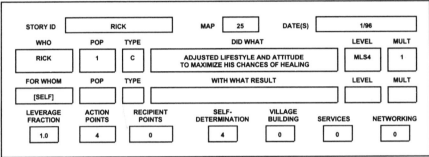

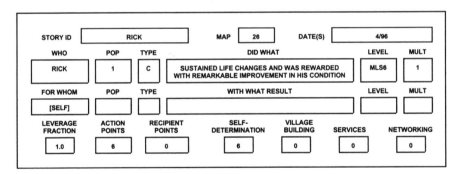

The last maps in the story (Maps 27–31) summarize Rick's recent activities as a motivational speaker (and village builder) for over 600 AIDS victims and their families. Since the period covered was 14 months, five maps were required. The service was ACT2→LEV2. Since data on actual numbers reached each three-month period were not provided, it was assumed that one-fifth or 120 were the recipients of each map.

| STORY ID | RICK | | MAP | 27 | DATE(S) | 7/96 TO 9/96 | |
|---|---|---|---|---|---|---|---|
| **WHO** | **POP** | **TYPE** | **DID WHAT** | | | **LEVEL** | **MULT** |
| RICK | 1 | VC | DELIVERED MOTIVATIONAL TALKS | | | ACT2 | 1 |
| **FOR WHOM** | **POP** | **TYPE** | **WITH WHAT RESULT** | | | **LEVEL** | **MULT** |
| AIDS VICTIMS | 120 | X | RECEIVED INSPIRATION AND ENCOURAGEMENT | | | LEV2 | 7 |

| LEVERAGE FRACTION | ACTION POINTS | RECIPIENT POINTS | SELF-DETERMINATION | VILLAGE BUILDING | SERVICES | NETWORKING |
|---|---|---|---|---|---|---|
| 1.0 | 2 | 14 | 0 | 2 | 14 | 0 |

| STORY ID | RICK | | MAP | 28 | DATE(S) | 10/96 TO 12/96 | |
|---|---|---|---|---|---|---|---|
| **WHO** | **POP** | **TYPE** | **DID WHAT** | | | **LEVEL** | **MULT** |
| RICK | 1 | VC | DELIVERED MOTIVATIONAL TALKS | | | ACT2 | 1 |
| **FOR WHOM** | **POP** | **TYPE** | **WITH WHAT RESULT** | | | **LEVEL** | **MULT** |
| AIDS VICTIMS | 120 | X | RECEIVED INSPIRATION AND ENCOURAGEMENT | | | LEV2 | 7 |

| LEVERAGE FRACTION | ACTION POINTS | RECIPIENT POINTS | SELF-DETERMINATION | VILLAGE BUILDING | SERVICES | NETWORKING |
|---|---|---|---|---|---|---|
| 1.0 | 2 | 14 | 0 | 2 | 14 | 0 |

| STORY ID | RICK | | MAP | 29 | DATE(S) | 1/97 TO 3/97 | |
|---|---|---|---|---|---|---|---|
| **WHO** | **POP** | **TYPE** | **DID WHAT** | | | **LEVEL** | **MULT** |
| RICK | 1 | VC | DELIVERED MOTIVATIONAL TALKS | | | ACT2 | 1 |
| **FOR WHOM** | **POP** | **TYPE** | **WITH WHAT RESULT** | | | **LEVEL** | **MULT** |
| AIDS VICTIMS | 120 | X | RECEIVED INSPIRATION AND ENCOURAGEMENT | | | LEV2 | 7 |

| LEVERAGE FRACTION | ACTION POINTS | RECIPIENT POINTS | SELF-DETERMINATION | VILLAGE BUILDING | SERVICES | NETWORKING |
|---|---|---|---|---|---|---|
| 1.0 | 2 | 14 | 0 | 2 | 14 | 0 |

| STORY ID | RICK | | MAP | 30 | DATE(S) | 4/97 TO 6/97 | |
|---|---|---|---|---|---|---|---|
| **WHO** | **POP** | **TYPE** | **DID WHAT** | | | **LEVEL** | **MULT** |
| RICK | 1 | VC | DELIVERED MOTIVATIONAL TALKS | | | ACT2 | 1 |
| **FOR WHOM** | **POP** | **TYPE** | **WITH WHAT RESULT** | | | **LEVEL** | **MULT** |
| AIDS VICTIMS | 120 | X | RECEIVED INSPIRATION AND ENCOURAGEMENT | | | LEV2 | 7 |

| LEVERAGE FRACTION | ACTION POINTS | RECIPIENT POINTS | SELF-DETERMINATION | VILLAGE BUILDING | SERVICES | NETWORKING |
|---|---|---|---|---|---|---|
| 1.0 | 2 | 14 | 0 | 2 | 14 | 0 |

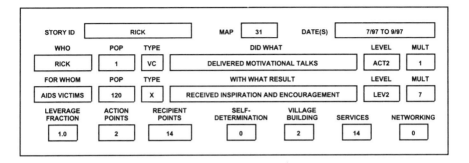

*Story Summary.* Rick's story earned the program 39 action points and 144 recipient points. Of the action points, 14 points represented self-determination (10 for Rick and 4 for his mother) and 25 points represented village building (15 by Jane in caring for her son and 10 for Rick in his activity as a motivational speaker). As earlier noted, none of the free services provided to Rick were considered acts of village building since the providers received salaries and grant funds covered other expenses. Of the recipient points, 48 points were for direct cl-I-ent services, 23 points were for services to a family member (i.e., to Jane), 8 points represented networking (from program staff to other local service providers), and the remaining 70 points reflected the "motivational impact" of Rick's presentations on the 600 persons who heard him speak (referred to as community member services). Program staff were the change agent in 13 of the 26 maps scored. Included were four handoffs (ACT2), three services directed at solving an immediate problem (ACT3), and six maps documenting sustained support and care (ACT5). Other local service providers were change agents in six of the 26 maps (five at ACT3 and one at ACT2). Jane was the change agent in four maps (three at ACT5 and one, for self-benefit, at MLS4). Rick was the change agent in the remaining seven maps (at MLS4, MLS6, and ACT2).

# STORY 3

The Pima Prevention Partnership (PPP) in Tucson, Arizona was established to promote healthy communities and reduce substance use and abuse among youth and adults in the city and surrounding county. In 1995, PPP staff spearheaded the creation of a community coalition to address over-representation of minority youth in the juvenile justice system. The coalition included Pima County Juvenile Court, Pima County Attorney's Office, Office of the Mayor, Pima County Justice

**Table 7.1.** Participation in Pima County Teen Court,
October 1995 to September 1997

| Period | Offenders | Adults | | | Youth | |
| | | Judges | Attorneys | Volunteers | Attorneys | Jurors |
|---|---|---|---|---|---|---|
| [2 years] | [120] | [9] | [45] | [27] | [42] | [93] |
| 10/95–12/95 | 24 | 4 | 8 | 6 | 10 | 26 |
| 1/96–3/96 | 24 | 4 | 9 | 8 | 10 | 29 |
| 4/96–6/96 | 30 | 6 | 7 | 8 | 10 | 32 |
| 7/96–9/96 | 30 | 5 | 12 | 10 | 15 | 40 |
| 10/96–12/96 | 40 | 6 | 12 | 11 | 15 | 53 |
| 1/97–3/97 | 40 | 7 | 14 | 15 | 13 | 51 |
| 4/97–6/97 | 30 | 8 | 11 | 15 | 15 | 42 |
| 7/97–9/97 | 22 | 6 | 7 | 11 | 10 | 38 |

Court, Pima County Bar Association, the Volunteer Center, the Metropolitan Education Commission, the Crime Prevention League, and members of several adult and youth grassroots coalitions.

In October 1995, the coalition launched the Pima County Teen Court. Teen Court is a sentencing proceeding and, as such, does not determine guilt or innocence. Eligible minors must agree to admit their guilt in open court and to complete the requirements of a sentence handed down by a jury of their peers. PPP staff and local social service agencies developed these sentencing options, which include a mandatory Teen Court Basic Training workshop, jury duty, letter of apology, and a range of prevention education workshops on life skills, communication, decision-making, anger management, and taking responsibility. Since its launching, 240 youth have appeared in Court with their parents and followed through with their sentencing. Of these, only 19 have been arrested for subsequent offenses.

Over the past two years, nine judges in Pima County have volunteered to preside over Teen Court on Saturday mornings at different times throughout the period. Forty-five members of the Pima County Bar have participated as coaches, trainers, and mentors to teen attorneys. Over 40 youth were trained to act as attorneys in the Teen Court. These youth have participated on a regular basis in weekly two-hour preparation workshops and five-hour Teen Court sessions. At least three lay adult volunteers have participated each Saturday at the Teen Court providing logistical and resource support for the parents of defendants and follow-up services to the family (a total of 27 adults in 1995–97). In addition, over 90 youth volunteered for jury duty (with these numbers supplemented by the defendants who later were required to serve on juries). Quarter-by-quarter counts of participants appear in Table 7.1.

It has been estimated that over 20,000 hours of community service—from defendants, teen and adult volunteers—have resulted. This ground-breaking ini-

**Table 7.2.** Numbers Trained for Pima County Teen Court,
Rounds One and Two

| Round | Dates | Adults | | | Youth | |
|---|---|---|---|---|---|---|
| | | Judges | Attorneys | Volunteers | Attorneys | Jurors |
| [2 years] | | [9] | [45] | [27] | [42] | [93] |
| Round 1 | 10/95–12/95 | 7 | 30 | 18 | 20 | 50 |
| Round 2 | 10/96–12/96 | 2 | 15 | 9 | 22 | 43 |

tiative served to open channels of communication and create trusting relationships among the coalition partners. Bolstered by the success of the Teen Court, members of the coalition have continued to work more closely with one another to create other significant shifts in the juvenile justice system.

From the outset, two staff persons from PPP have assumed primary responsibility for the workings of Teen Court. They oversee recruitment, assignment of tasks, training, sentencing programs, and coalition maintenance activities. There were two rounds of training during which participants were recruited and trained. The first round took place between October and December 1995; the second round took place one year later (October to December 1996). Table 7.2 indicates the numbers trained, by role played in the Court. Most of the first-round participants continued to participate during the second year as well.

Unlike the first two stories, the Teen Court story is not mapped at the personal level. Rather, the various participants are grouped according to the services provided or the benefits received.

# Story 3 Mapped

Again, Map 0 is used to provide the context.

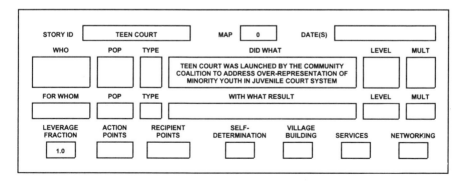

The primary cl-I-ents of this story are the 240 youth who were allowed to appear in Teen Court for sentencing rather than be subjected to the juvenile court system. However, since Teen Court was also intended from the outset as a primary prevention activity to support and encourage active involvement by youth in civic affairs, all the youth in the story were considered cl-I-ents.

Maps 1 and 2 depict the recruitment and training of the first groups of 20 attorneys and 50 jury members in the first quarter (October to December 1995). They are mapped separately, since each group received specialized training at different times.

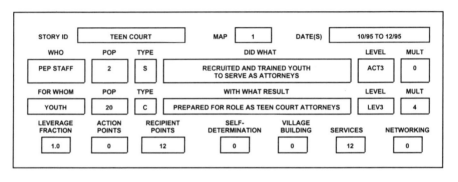

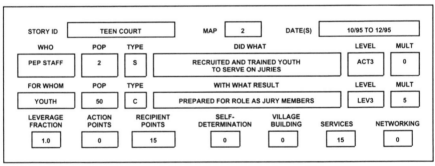

The next three maps (Maps 3–5) document the first-round recruitment and preparation for Court activities of the judges, professional attorneys, and adult volunteers. The judges and attorneys were also considered volunteers in later maps when they were the change agents.

| STORY ID | TEEN COURT | | MAP | 3 | DATE(S) | 10/95 TO 12/95 | |
|---|---|---|---|---|---|---|---|

| WHO | POP | TYPE | DID WHAT | | | LEVEL | MULT |
|---|---|---|---|---|---|---|---|
| PEP STAFF | 2 | S | RECRUITED AND PREPARED JUDGES | | | ACT3 | 0 |

| FOR WHOM | POP | TYPE | WITH WHAT RESULT | | | LEVEL | MULT |
|---|---|---|---|---|---|---|---|
| JUDGES | 7 | P | PREPARED FOR ROLE AS TEEN COURT JUDGES | | | LEV3 | 3 |

| LEVERAGE FRACTION | ACTION POINTS | RECIPIENT POINTS | SELF-DETERMINATION | VILLAGE BUILDING | SERVICES | NETWORKING |
|---|---|---|---|---|---|---|
| 1.0 | 0 | 9 | 0 | 0 | 9 | 0 |

| STORY ID | TEEN COURT | | MAP | 4 | DATE(S) | 10/95 TO 12/95 | |
|---|---|---|---|---|---|---|---|

| WHO | POP | TYPE | DID WHAT | | | LEVEL | MULT |
|---|---|---|---|---|---|---|---|
| PEP STAFF | 2 | S | RECRUITED AND PREPARED ATTORNEYS | | | ACT3 | 0 |

| FOR WHOM | POP | TYPE | WITH WHAT RESULT | | | LEVEL | MULT |
|---|---|---|---|---|---|---|---|
| ATTORNEYS | 30 | P | PREPARED TO SERVE AS COACHES AND MENTORS | | | LEV3 | 5 |

| LEVERAGE FRACTION | ACTION POINTS | RECIPIENT POINTS | SELF-DETERMINATION | VILLAGE BUILDING | SERVICES | NETWORKING |
|---|---|---|---|---|---|---|
| 1.0 | 0 | 15 | 0 | 0 | 15 | 0 |

| STORY ID | TEEN COURT | | MAP | 5 | DATE(S) | 10/95 TO 12/95 | |
|---|---|---|---|---|---|---|---|

| WHO | POP | TYPE | DID WHAT | | | LEVEL | MULT |
|---|---|---|---|---|---|---|---|
| PEP STAFF | 2 | S | RECRUITED AND TRAINED VOLUNTEERS | | | ACT3 | 0 |

| FOR WHOM | POP | TYPE | WITH WHAT RESULT | | | LEVEL | MULT |
|---|---|---|---|---|---|---|---|
| ADULTS | 18 | X | PREPARED FOR VARIOUS ROLES IN SUPPORT OF PARENTS OF DEFENDANTS | | | LEV3 | 4 |

| LEVERAGE FRACTION | ACTION POINTS | RECIPIENT POINTS | SELF-DETERMINATION | VILLAGE BUILDING | SERVICES | NETWORKING |
|---|---|---|---|---|---|---|
| 1.0 | 0 | 12 | 0 | 0 | 12 | 0 |

Maps 6 through 9 document the ongoing coaching and training provided by the 30 professional attorneys to the 20 teen attorneys throughout the first year. The actual numbers involved each quarter were obtained from Table 7.1 in the narrative.

| STORY ID | TEEN COURT | | MAP | 6 | DATE(S) | | 10/95 TO 12/95 | |
|---|---|---|---|---|---|---|---|---|
| WHO | POP | TYPE | DID WHAT | | | | LEVEL | MULT |
| ATTORNEYS | 8 | VP | PREPARED TEEN ATTORNEYS FOR THEIR ROLE | | | | ACT3 | 3 |
| FOR WHOM | POP | TYPE | WITH WHAT RESULT | | | | LEVEL | MULT |
| YOUTH | 10 | C | PREPARED FOR THEIR KEY ROLE IN THE COURT | | | | LEV3 | 3 |

| LEVERAGE FRACTION | ACTION POINTS | RECIPIENT POINTS | SELF-DETERMINATION | VILLAGE BUILDING | SERVICES | NETWORKING |
|---|---|---|---|---|---|---|
| 1.0 | 9 | 9 | 0 | 9 | 9 | 0 |

| STORY ID | TEEN COURT | | MAP | 7 | DATE(S) | | 1/96 TO 3/96 | |
|---|---|---|---|---|---|---|---|---|
| WHO | POP | TYPE | DID WHAT | | | | LEVEL | MULT |
| ATTORNEYS | 9 | VP | PREPARED TEEN ATTORNEYS FOR THEIR ROLE | | | | ACT3 | 3 |
| FOR WHOM | POP | TYPE | WITH WHAT RESULT | | | | LEVEL | MULT |
| YOUTH | 10 | C | PREPARED FOR THEIR KEY ROLE IN THE COURT | | | | LEV3 | 3 |

| LEVERAGE FRACTION | ACTION POINTS | RECIPIENT POINTS | SELF-DETERMINATION | VILLAGE BUILDING | SERVICES | NETWORKING |
|---|---|---|---|---|---|---|
| 1.0 | 9 | 9 | 0 | 9 | 9 | 0 |

| STORY ID | TEEN COURT | | MAP | 8 | DATE(S) | | 4/96 TO 6/96 | |
|---|---|---|---|---|---|---|---|---|
| WHO | POP | TYPE | DID WHAT | | | | LEVEL | MULT |
| ATTORNEYS | 7 | VP | PREPARED TEEN ATTORNEYS FOR THEIR ROLE | | | | ACT3 | 3 |
| FOR WHOM | POP | TYPE | WITH WHAT RESULT | | | | LEVEL | MULT |
| YOUTH | 10 | C | PREPARED FOR THEIR KEY ROLE IN THE COURT | | | | LEV3 | 3 |

| LEVERAGE FRACTION | ACTION POINTS | RECIPIENT POINTS | SELF-DETERMINATION | VILLAGE BUILDING | SERVICES | NETWORKING |
|---|---|---|---|---|---|---|
| 1.0 | 9 | 9 | 0 | 9 | 9 | 0 |

| STORY ID | TEEN COURT | | MAP | 9 | DATE(S) | | 7/96 TO 9/96 | |
|---|---|---|---|---|---|---|---|---|
| WHO | POP | TYPE | DID WHAT | | | | LEVEL | MULT |
| ATTORNEYS | 12 | VP | PREPARED TEEN ATTORNEYS FOR THEIR ROLE | | | | ACT3 | 4 |
| FOR WHOM | POP | TYPE | WITH WHAT RESULT | | | | LEVEL | MULT |
| YOUTH | 15 | C | PREPARED FOR THEIR KEY ROLE IN THE COURT | | | | LEV3 | 4 |

| LEVERAGE FRACTION | ACTION POINTS | RECIPIENT POINTS | SELF-DETERMINATION | VILLAGE BUILDING | SERVICES | NETWORKING |
|---|---|---|---|---|---|---|
| 1.0 | 12 | 12 | 0 | 12 | 12 | 0 |

Split maps (Maps 10a, b, c through 13a, b, c) cover the actual court proceedings during the first year. The change agents are the judges, teen attorneys, and teen jurors. The recipients are the teen defendants. By convention, the latter appear in only the first map of each set. Since the teen attorneys and jury members were considered cl-I-ents (who were learning and growing through this process), their actions were coded as self-determination rather than as village building—though either code would apply.

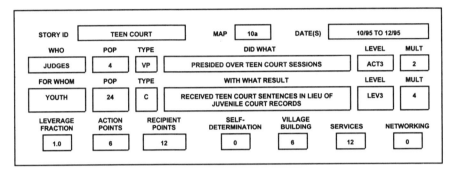

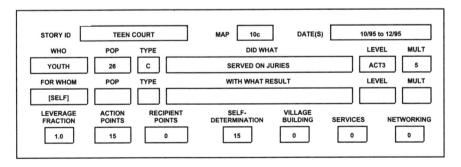

| STORY ID | TEEN COURT | | MAP | 11a | DATE(S) | 1/96 TO 3/96 | |
|---|---|---|---|---|---|---|---|
| WHO | POP | TYPE | | DID WHAT | | LEVEL | MULT |
| JUDGES | 4 | VP | PRESIDED OVER TEEN COURT SESSIONS | | | ACT3 | 2 |
| FOR WHOM | POP | TYPE | | WITH WHAT RESULT | | LEVEL | MULT |
| YOUTH | 24 | C | RECEIVED TEEN COURT SENTENCES IN LIEU OF JUVENILE COURT RECORDS | | | LEV3 | 4 |
| LEVERAGE FRACTION | ACTION POINTS | RECIPIENT POINTS | SELF-DETERMINATION | VILLAGE BUILDING | SERVICES | NETWORKING | |
| 1.0 | 6 | 12 | 0 | 6 | 12 | 0 | |

| STORY ID | TEEN COURT | | MAP | 11b | DATE(S) | 1/96 TO 3/96 | |
|---|---|---|---|---|---|---|---|
| WHO | POP | TYPE | | DID WHAT | | LEVEL | MULT |
| YOUTH | 10 | C | SERVED AS ATTORNEYS | | | ACT3 | 3 |
| FOR WHOM | POP | TYPE | | WITH WHAT RESULT | | LEVEL | MULT |
| [SELF] | | | | | | | |
| LEVERAGE FRACTION | ACTION POINTS | RECIPIENT POINTS | SELF-DETERMINATION | VILLAGE BUILDING | SERVICES | NETWORKING | |
| 1.0 | 9 | 0 | 9 | 0 | 0 | 0 | |

| STORY ID | TEEN COURT | | MAP | 11c | DATE(S) | 1/96 TO 3/96 | |
|---|---|---|---|---|---|---|---|
| WHO | POP | TYPE | | DID WHAT | | LEVEL | MULT |
| YOUTH | 29 | C | SERVED ON JURIES | | | ACT3 | 5 |
| FOR WHOM | POP | TYPE | | WITH WHAT RESULT | | LEVEL | MULT |
| [SELF] | | | | | | | |
| LEVERAGE FRACTION | ACTION POINTS | RECIPIENT POINTS | SELF-DETERMINATION | VILLAGE BUILDING | SERVICES | NETWORKING | |
| 1.0 | 15 | 0 | 15 | 0 | 0 | 0 | |

| STORY ID | TEEN COURT | | MAP | 12a | DATE(S) | 4/96 TO 6/96 | |
|---|---|---|---|---|---|---|---|
| WHO | POP | TYPE | | DID WHAT | | LEVEL | MULT |
| JUDGES | 6 | VP | PRESIDED OVER TEEN COURT SESSIONS | | | ACT3 | 3 |
| FOR WHOM | POP | TYPE | | WITH WHAT RESULT | | LEVEL | MULT |
| YOUTH | 30 | C | RECEIVED TEEN COURT SENTENCES IN LIEU OF JUVENILE COURT RECORDS | | | LEV3 | 5 |
| LEVERAGE FRACTION | ACTION POINTS | RECIPIENT POINTS | SELF-DETERMINATION | VILLAGE BUILDING | SERVICES | NETWORKING | |
| 1.0 | 9 | 15 | 0 | 9 | 15 | 0 | |

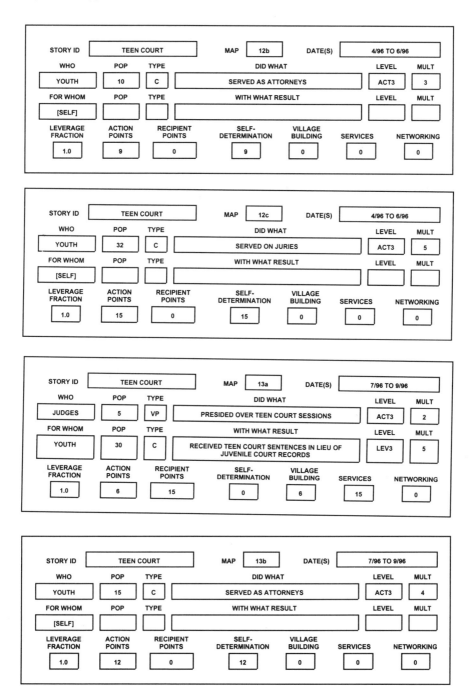

| STORY ID | TEEN COURT | | MAP | 13c | DATE(S) | 7/96 TO 9/96 | |
|---|---|---|---|---|---|---|---|
| WHO | POP | TYPE | DID WHAT | | | LEVEL | MULT |
| YOUTH | 40 | C | SERVED ON JURIES | | | ACT3 | 5 |
| FOR WHOM | POP | TYPE | WITH WHAT RESULT | | | LEVEL | MULT |
| [SELF] | | | | | | | |
| LEVERAGE FRACTION | ACTION POINTS | RECIPIENT POINTS | SELF-DETERMINATION | VILLAGE BUILDING | SERVICES | | NETWORKING |
| 1.0 | 15 | 0 | 15 | 0 | 0 | | 0 |

The next set of maps (Maps 14–17) covers the role played by the adult volunteers in supporting the parents of the defendants (the number of parents was estimated at 40 each quarter based on the number of offenders).

| STORY ID | TEEN COURT | | MAP | 14 | DATE(S) | 10/95 TO 12/95 | |
|---|---|---|---|---|---|---|---|
| WHO | POP | TYPE | DID WHAT | | | LEVEL | MULT |
| ADULTS | 6 | VX | SUPPORTED NEEDS OF PARENTS OF DEFENDANTS | | | ACT3 | 3 |
| FOR WHOM | POP | TYPE | WITH WHAT RESULT | | | LEVEL | MULT |
| PARENTS | 40 | F | RECEIVED VARIOUS SERVICES AND SUPPORT | | | LEV3 | 5 |
| LEVERAGE FRACTION | ACTION POINTS | RECIPIENT POINTS | SELF-DETERMINATION | VILLAGE BUILDING | SERVICES | | NETWORKING |
| 1.0 | 9 | 15 | 0 | 9 | 15 | | 0 |

| STORY ID | TEEN COURT | | MAP | 15 | DATE(S) | 1/96 TO 3/96 | |
|---|---|---|---|---|---|---|---|
| WHO | POP | TYPE | DID WHAT | | | LEVEL | MULT |
| ADULTS | 8 | VX | SUPPORTED NEEDS OF PARENTS OF DEFENDANTS | | | ACT3 | 3 |
| FOR WHOM | POP | TYPE | WITH WHAT RESULT | | | LEVEL | MULT |
| PARENTS | 40 | F | RECEIVED VARIOUS SERVICES AND SUPPORT | | | LEV3 | 5 |
| LEVERAGE FRACTION | ACTION POINTS | RECIPIENT POINTS | SELF-DETERMINATION | VILLAGE BUILDING | SERVICES | | NETWORKING |
| 1.0 | 9 | 15 | 0 | 9 | 15 | | 0 |

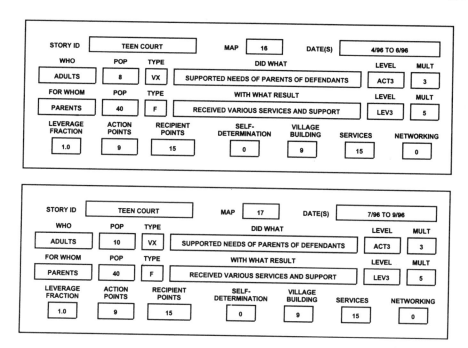

This complete set of 17 maps was repeated for the second year of the Court (i.e., from October 1996 through September 1997). The maps were near identical; only the dates changed, and the counts of offenders and participants each quarter.

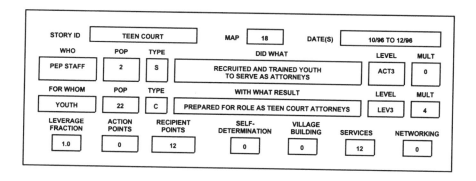

| STORY ID | TEEN COURT | | | MAP | 19 | DATE(S) | 10/96 TO 12/96 | |
|---|---|---|---|---|---|---|---|---|

| WHO | POP | TYPE | DID WHAT | LEVEL | MULT |
|---|---|---|---|---|---|
| PEP STAFF | 2 | S | RECRUITED AND TRAINED YOUTH TO SERVE ON JURIES | ACT3 | 0 |

| FOR WHOM | POP | TYPE | WITH WHAT RESULT | LEVEL | MULT |
|---|---|---|---|---|---|
| YOUTH | 43 | C | PREPARED FOR ROLE AS JURY MEMBERS | LEV3 | 5 |

| LEVERAGE FRACTION | ACTION POINTS | RECIPIENT POINTS | SELF-DETERMINATION | VILLAGE BUILDING | SERVICES | NETWORKING |
|---|---|---|---|---|---|---|
| 1.0 | 0 | 15 | 0 | 0 | 15 | 0 |

| STORY ID | TEEN COURT | | | MAP | 20 | DATE(S) | 10/96 TO 12/96 | |
|---|---|---|---|---|---|---|---|---|

| WHO | POP | TYPE | DID WHAT | LEVEL | MULT |
|---|---|---|---|---|---|
| PEP STAFF | 2 | S | RECRUITED AND PREPARED JUDGES | ACT3 | 0 |

| FOR WHOM | POP | TYPE | WITH WHAT RESULT | LEVEL | MULT |
|---|---|---|---|---|---|
| JUDGES | 2 | P | PREPARED FOR ROLE AS TEEN COURT JUDGES | LEV3 | 2 |

| LEVERAGE FRACTION | ACTION POINTS | RECIPIENT POINTS | SELF-DETERMINATION | VILLAGE BUILDING | SERVICES | NETWORKING |
|---|---|---|---|---|---|---|
| 1.0 | 0 | 6 | 0 | 0 | 6 | 0 |

| STORY ID | TEEN COURT | | | MAP | 21 | DATE(S) | 10/96 TO 12/96 | |
|---|---|---|---|---|---|---|---|---|

| WHO | POP | TYPE | DID WHAT | LEVEL | MULT |
|---|---|---|---|---|---|
| PEP STAFF | 2 | S | RECRUITED AND PREPARED ATTORNEYS | ACT3 | 0 |

| FOR WHOM | POP | TYPE | WITH WHAT RESULT | LEVEL | MULT |
|---|---|---|---|---|---|
| ATTORNEYS | 15 | P | PREPARED TO SERVE AS COACHES AND MENTORS | LEV3 | 5 |

| LEVERAGE FRACTION | ACTION POINTS | RECIPIENT POINTS | SELF-DETERMINATION | VILLAGE BUILDING | SERVICES | NETWORKING |
|---|---|---|---|---|---|---|
| 1.0 | 0 | 12 | 0 | 0 | 12 | 0 |

| STORY ID | TEEN COURT | | | MAP | 22 | DATE(S) | 10/96 TO 12/96 | |
|---|---|---|---|---|---|---|---|---|

| WHO | POP | TYPE | DID WHAT | LEVEL | MULT |
|---|---|---|---|---|---|
| PEP STAFF | 2 | S | RECRUITED AND TRAINED VOLUNTEERS | ACT3 | 0 |

| FOR WHOM | POP | TYPE | WITH WHAT RESULT | LEVEL | MULT |
|---|---|---|---|---|---|
| ADULTS | 9 | X | PREPARED FOR VARIOUS ROLES IN SUPPORT OF PARENTS OF DEFENDANTS | LEV3 | 3 |

| LEVERAGE FRACTION | ACTION POINTS | RECIPIENT POINTS | SELF-DETERMINATION | VILLAGE BUILDING | SERVICES | NETWORKING |
|---|---|---|---|---|---|---|
| 1.0 | 0 | 9 | 0 | 0 | 9 | 0 |

| STORY ID | TEEN COURT | MAP | 23 | DATE(S) | 10/96 TO 12/96 |
|---|---|---|---|---|---|

| WHO | POP | TYPE | DID WHAT | LEVEL | MULT |
|---|---|---|---|---|---|
| ATTORNEYS | 12 | VP | PREPARED TEEN ATTORNEYS FOR THEIR ROLE | ACT3 | 4 |

| FOR WHOM | POP | TYPE | WITH WHAT RESULT | LEVEL | MULT |
|---|---|---|---|---|---|
| YOUTH | 15 | C | PREPARED FOR THEIR KEY ROLE IN THE COURT | LEV3 | 4 |

| LEVERAGE FRACTION | ACTION POINTS | RECIPIENT POINTS | SELF-DETERMINATION | VILLAGE BUILDING | SERVICES | NETWORKING |
|---|---|---|---|---|---|---|
| 1.0 | 12 | 12 | 0 | 12 | 12 | 0 |

| STORY ID | TEEN COURT | MAP | 24 | DATE(S) | 1/97 TO 3/97 |
|---|---|---|---|---|---|

| WHO | POP | TYPE | DID WHAT | LEVEL | MULT |
|---|---|---|---|---|---|
| ATTORNEYS | 14 | VP | PREPARED TEEN ATTORNEYS FOR THEIR ROLE | ACT3 | 4 |

| FOR WHOM | POP | TYPE | WITH WHAT RESULT | LEVEL | MULT |
|---|---|---|---|---|---|
| YOUTH | 13 | C | PREPARED FOR THEIR KEY ROLE IN THE COURT | LEV3 | 4 |

| LEVERAGE FRACTION | ACTION POINTS | RECIPIENT POINTS | SELF-DETERMINATION | VILLAGE BUILDING | SERVICES | NETWORKING |
|---|---|---|---|---|---|---|
| 1.0 | 12 | 12 | 0 | 12 | 12 | 0 |

| STORY ID | TEEN COURT | MAP | 25 | DATE(S) | 4/97 TO 6/97 |
|---|---|---|---|---|---|

| WHO | POP | TYPE | DID WHAT | LEVEL | MULT |
|---|---|---|---|---|---|
| ATTORNEYS | 11 | VP | PREPARED TEEN ATTORNEYS FOR THEIR ROLE | ACT3 | 4 |

| FOR WHOM | POP | TYPE | WITH WHAT RESULT | LEVEL | MULT |
|---|---|---|---|---|---|
| YOUTH | 15 | C | PREPARED FOR THEIR KEY ROLE IN THE COURT | LEV3 | 4 |

| LEVERAGE FRACTION | ACTION POINTS | RECIPIENT POINTS | SELF-DETERMINATION | VILLAGE BUILDING | SERVICES | NETWORKING |
|---|---|---|---|---|---|---|
| 1.0 | 12 | 12 | 0 | 12 | 12 | 0 |

| STORY ID | TEEN COURT | MAP | 26 | DATE(S) | 7/97 TO 9/97 |
|---|---|---|---|---|---|

| WHO | POP | TYPE | DID WHAT | LEVEL | MULT |
|---|---|---|---|---|---|
| ATTORNEYS | 7 | VP | PREPARED TEEN ATTORNEYS FOR THEIR ROLE | ACT3 | 3 |

| FOR WHOM | POP | TYPE | WITH WHAT RESULT | LEVEL | MULT |
|---|---|---|---|---|---|
| YOUTH | 10 | C | PREPARED FOR THEIR KEY ROLE IN THE COURT | LEV3 | 3 |

| LEVERAGE FRACTION | ACTION POINTS | RECIPIENT POINTS | SELF-DETERMINATION | VILLAGE BUILDING | SERVICES | NETWORKING |
|---|---|---|---|---|---|---|
| 1.0 | 9 | 9 | 0 | 9 | 9 | 0 |

| STORY ID | TEEN COURT | | | MAP | 27a | DATE(S) | 10/96 TO 12/96 | |
|---|---|---|---|---|---|---|---|---|

| WHO | POP | TYPE | DID WHAT | LEVEL | MULT |
|---|---|---|---|---|---|
| JUDGES | 6 | VP | PRESIDED OVER TEEN COURT SESSIONS | ACT3 | 3 |

| FOR WHOM | POP | TYPE | WITH WHAT RESULT | LEVEL | MULT |
|---|---|---|---|---|---|
| YOUTH | 40 | C | RECEIVED TEEN COURT SENTENCES IN LIEU OF JUVENILE COURT RECORDS | LEV3 | 5 |

| LEVERAGE FRACTION | ACTION POINTS | RECIPIENT POINTS | SELF-DETERMINATION | VILLAGE BUILDING | SERVICES | NETWORKING |
|---|---|---|---|---|---|---|
| 1.0 | 9 | 15 | 0 | 9 | 15 | 0 |

| STORY ID | TEEN COURT | | | MAP | 27b | DATE(S) | 10/96 to 12/96 | |
|---|---|---|---|---|---|---|---|---|

| WHO | POP | TYPE | DID WHAT | LEVEL | MULT |
|---|---|---|---|---|---|
| YOUTH | 15 | C | SERVED AS ATTORNEYS | ACT3 | 4 |

| FOR WHOM | POP | TYPE | WITH WHAT RESULT | LEVEL | MULT |
|---|---|---|---|---|---|
| [SELF] | | | | | |

| LEVERAGE FRACTION | ACTION POINTS | RECIPIENT POINTS | SELF-DETERMINATION | VILLAGE BUILDING | SERVICES | NETWORKING |
|---|---|---|---|---|---|---|
| 1.0 | 12 | 0 | 12 | 0 | 0 | 0 |

| STORY ID | TEEN COURT | | | MAP | 27c | DATE(S) | 10/96 to 12/96 | |
|---|---|---|---|---|---|---|---|---|

| WHO | POP | TYPE | DID WHAT | LEVEL | MULT |
|---|---|---|---|---|---|
| YOUTH | 53 | C | SERVED ON JURIES | ACT3 | 6 |

| FOR WHOM | POP | TYPE | WITH WHAT RESULT | LEVEL | MULT |
|---|---|---|---|---|---|
| [SELF] | | | | | |

| LEVERAGE FRACTION | ACTION POINTS | RECIPIENT POINTS | SELF-DETERMINATION | VILLAGE BUILDING | SERVICES | NETWORKING |
|---|---|---|---|---|---|---|
| 1.0 | 18 | 0 | 18 | 0 | 0 | 0 |

| STORY ID | TEEN COURT | | | MAP | 28a | DATE(S) | 1/97 TO 3/97 | |
|---|---|---|---|---|---|---|---|---|

| WHO | POP | TYPE | DID WHAT | LEVEL | MULT |
|---|---|---|---|---|---|
| JUDGES | 7 | VP | PRESIDED OVER TEEN COURT SESSIONS | ACT3 | 3 |

| FOR WHOM | POP | TYPE | WITH WHAT RESULT | LEVEL | MULT |
|---|---|---|---|---|---|
| YOUTH | 40 | C | RECEIVED TEEN COURT SENTENCES IN LIEU OF JUVENILE COURT RECORDS | LEV3 | 5 |

| LEVERAGE FRACTION | ACTION POINTS | RECIPIENT POINTS | SELF-DETERMINATION | VILLAGE BUILDING | SERVICES | NETWORKING |
|---|---|---|---|---|---|---|
| 1.0 | 9 | 15 | 0 | 9 | 15 | 0 |

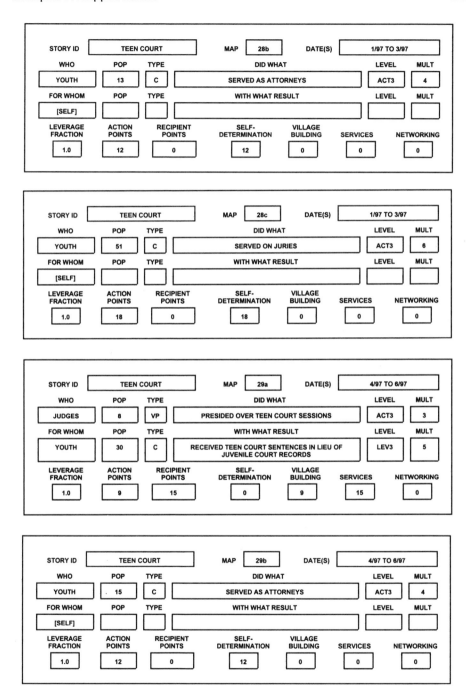

| STORY ID | TEEN COURT | | MAP | 28b | DATE(S) | 1/97 TO 3/97 |
|---|---|---|---|---|---|---|

| WHO | POP | TYPE | DID WHAT | LEVEL | MULT |
|---|---|---|---|---|---|
| YOUTH | 13 | C | SERVED AS ATTORNEYS | ACT3 | 4 |

| FOR WHOM | POP | TYPE | WITH WHAT RESULT | LEVEL | MULT |
|---|---|---|---|---|---|
| [SELF] | | | | | |

| LEVERAGE FRACTION | ACTION POINTS | RECIPIENT POINTS | SELF-DETERMINATION | VILLAGE BUILDING | SERVICES | NETWORKING |
|---|---|---|---|---|---|---|
| 1.0 | 12 | 0 | 12 | 0 | 0 | 0 |


| STORY ID | TEEN COURT | | MAP | 28c | DATE(S) | 1/97 TO 3/97 |
|---|---|---|---|---|---|---|

| WHO | POP | TYPE | DID WHAT | LEVEL | MULT |
|---|---|---|---|---|---|
| YOUTH | 51 | C | SERVED ON JURIES | ACT3 | 6 |

| FOR WHOM | POP | TYPE | WITH WHAT RESULT | LEVEL | MULT |
|---|---|---|---|---|---|
| [SELF] | | | | | |

| LEVERAGE FRACTION | ACTION POINTS | RECIPIENT POINTS | SELF-DETERMINATION | VILLAGE BUILDING | SERVICES | NETWORKING |
|---|---|---|---|---|---|---|
| 1.0 | 18 | 0 | 18 | 0 | 0 | 0 |


| STORY ID | TEEN COURT | | MAP | 29a | DATE(S) | 4/97 TO 6/97 |
|---|---|---|---|---|---|---|

| WHO | POP | TYPE | DID WHAT | LEVEL | MULT |
|---|---|---|---|---|---|
| JUDGES | 8 | VP | PRESIDED OVER TEEN COURT SESSIONS | ACT3 | 3 |

| FOR WHOM | POP | TYPE | WITH WHAT RESULT | LEVEL | MULT |
|---|---|---|---|---|---|
| YOUTH | 30 | C | RECEIVED TEEN COURT SENTENCES IN LIEU OF JUVENILE COURT RECORDS | LEV3 | 5 |

| LEVERAGE FRACTION | ACTION POINTS | RECIPIENT POINTS | SELF-DETERMINATION | VILLAGE BUILDING | SERVICES | NETWORKING |
|---|---|---|---|---|---|---|
| 1.0 | 9 | 15 | 0 | 9 | 15 | 0 |


| STORY ID | TEEN COURT | | MAP | 29b | DATE(S) | 4/97 TO 6/97 |
|---|---|---|---|---|---|---|

| WHO | POP | TYPE | DID WHAT | LEVEL | MULT |
|---|---|---|---|---|---|
| YOUTH | . 15 | C | SERVED AS ATTORNEYS | ACT3 | 4 |

| FOR WHOM | POP | TYPE | WITH WHAT RESULT | LEVEL | MULT |
|---|---|---|---|---|---|
| [SELF] | | | | | |

| LEVERAGE FRACTION | ACTION POINTS | RECIPIENT POINTS | SELF-DETERMINATION | VILLAGE BUILDING | SERVICES | NETWORKING |
|---|---|---|---|---|---|---|
| 1.0 | 12 | 0 | 12 | 0 | 0 | 0 |

| STORY ID | TEEN COURT | | MAP | 29c | DATE(S) | 4/97 TO 6/97 |
|---|---|---|---|---|---|---|

| WHO | POP | TYPE | DID WHAT | LEVEL | MULT |
|---|---|---|---|---|---|
| YOUTH | 42 | C | SERVED ON JURIES | ACT3 | 5 |

| FOR WHOM | POP | TYPE | WITH WHAT RESULT | LEVEL | MULT |
|---|---|---|---|---|---|
| [SELF] | | | | | |

| LEVERAGE FRACTION | ACTION POINTS | RECIPIENT POINTS | SELF-DETERMINATION | VILLAGE BUILDING | SERVICES | NETWORKING |
|---|---|---|---|---|---|---|
| 1.0 | 15 | 0 | 15 | 0 | 0 | 0 |

---

| STORY ID | TEEN COURT | | MAP | 30a | DATE(S) | 7/97 TO 9/97 |
|---|---|---|---|---|---|---|

| WHO | POP | TYPE | DID WHAT | LEVEL | MULT |
|---|---|---|---|---|---|
| JUDGES | 6 | VP | PRESIDED OVER TEEN COURT SESSIONS | ACT3 | 3 |

| FOR WHOM | POP | TYPE | WITH WHAT RESULT | LEVEL | MULT |
|---|---|---|---|---|---|
| YOUTH | 22 | C | RECEIVED TEEN COURT SENTENCES IN LIEU OF JUVENILE COURT RECORDS | LEV3 | 4 |

| LEVERAGE FRACTION | ACTION POINTS | RECIPIENT POINTS | SELF-DETERMINATION | VILLAGE BUILDING | SERVICES | NETWORKING |
|---|---|---|---|---|---|---|
| 1.0 | 9 | 12 | 0 | 9 | 12 | 0 |

---

| STORY ID | TEEN COURT | | MAP | 30b | DATE(S) | 7/97 TO 9/97 |
|---|---|---|---|---|---|---|

| WHO | POP | TYPE | DID WHAT | LEVEL | MULT |
|---|---|---|---|---|---|
| YOUTH | 10 | C | SERVED AS ATTORNEYS | ACT3 | 3 |

| FOR WHOM | POP | TYPE | WITH WHAT RESULT | LEVEL | MULT |
|---|---|---|---|---|---|
| [SELF] | | | | | |

| LEVERAGE FRACTION | ACTION POINTS | RECIPIENT POINTS | SELF-DETERMINATION | VILLAGE BUILDING | SERVICES | NETWORKING |
|---|---|---|---|---|---|---|
| 1.0 | 9 | 0 | 9 | 0 | 0 | 0 |

---

| STORY ID | TEEN COURT | | MAP | 30c | DATE(S) | 7/97 TO 9/97 |
|---|---|---|---|---|---|---|

| WHO | POP | TYPE | DID WHAT | LEVEL | MULT |
|---|---|---|---|---|---|
| YOUTH | 38 | C | SERVED ON JURIES | ACT3 | 5 |

| FOR WHOM | POP | TYPE | WITH WHAT RESULT | LEVEL | MULT |
|---|---|---|---|---|---|
| [SELF] | | | | | |

| LEVERAGE FRACTION | ACTION POINTS | RECIPIENT POINTS | SELF-DETERMINATION | VILLAGE BUILDING | SERVICES | NETWORKING |
|---|---|---|---|---|---|---|
| 1.0 | 15 | 0 | 15 | 0 | 0 | 0 |

| STORY ID | TEEN COURT | | MAP | 31 | DATE(S) | 10/96 TO 12/96 | |
|---|---|---|---|---|---|---|---|
| WHO | POP | TYPE | DID WHAT | | | LEVEL | MULT |
| ADULTS | 11 | VX | SUPPORTED NEEDS OF PARENTS OF DEFENDANTS | | | ACT3 | 4 |
| FOR WHOM | POP | TYPE | WITH WHAT RESULT | | | LEVEL | MULT |
| PARENTS | 40 | F | RECEIVED VARIOUS SERVICES AND SUPPORT | | | LEV3 | 5 |

| LEVERAGE FRACTION | ACTION POINTS | RECIPIENT POINTS | SELF-DETERMINATION | VILLAGE BUILDING | SERVICES | NETWORKING |
|---|---|---|---|---|---|---|
| 1.0 | 12 | 15 | 0 | 12 | 15 | 0 |

| STORY ID | TEEN COURT | | MAP | 32 | DATE(S) | 1/97 TO 3/97 | |
|---|---|---|---|---|---|---|---|
| WHO | POP | TYPE | DID WHAT | | | LEVEL | MULT |
| ADULTS | 15 | VX | SUPPORTED NEEDS OF PARENTS OF DEFENDANTS | | | ACT3 | 4 |
| FOR WHOM | POP | TYPE | WITH WHAT RESULT | | | LEVEL | MULT |
| PARENTS | 40 | F | RECEIVED VARIOUS SERVICES AND SUPPORT | | | LEV3 | 5 |

| LEVERAGE FRACTION | ACTION POINTS | RECIPIENT POINTS | SELF-DETERMINATION | VILLAGE BUILDING | SERVICES | NETWORKING |
|---|---|---|---|---|---|---|
| 1.0 | 12 | 15 | 0 | 12 | 15 | 0 |

| STORY ID | TEEN COURT | | MAP | 33 | DATE(S) | 4/97 TO 6/97 | |
|---|---|---|---|---|---|---|---|
| WHO | POP | TYPE | DID WHAT | | | LEVEL | MULT |
| ADULTS | 15 | VX | SUPPORTED NEEDS OF PARENTS OF DEFENDANTS | | | ACT3 | 4 |
| FOR WHOM | POP | TYPE | WITH WHAT RESULT | | | LEVEL | MULT |
| PARENTS | 40 | F | RECEIVED VARIOUS SERVICES AND SUPPORT | | | LEV3 | 5 |

| LEVERAGE FRACTION | ACTION POINTS | RECIPIENT POINTS | SELF-DETERMINATION | VILLAGE BUILDING | SERVICES | NETWORKING |
|---|---|---|---|---|---|---|
| 1.0 | 12 | 15 | 0 | 12 | 15 | 0 |

| STORY ID | TEEN COURT | | MAP | 34 | DATE(S) | 7/97 TO 9/97 | |
|---|---|---|---|---|---|---|---|
| WHO | POP | TYPE | DID WHAT | | | LEVEL | MULT |
| ADULTS | 11 | VX | SUPPORTED NEEDS OF PARENTS OF DEFENDANTS | | | ACT3 | 4 |
| FOR WHOM | POP | TYPE | WITH WHAT RESULT | | | LEVEL | MULT |
| PARENTS | 40 | F | RECEIVED VARIOUS SERVICES AND SUPPORT | | | LEV3 | 5 |

| LEVERAGE FRACTION | ACTION POINTS | RECIPIENT POINTS | SELF-DETERMINATION | VILLAGE BUILDING | SERVICES | NETWORKING |
|---|---|---|---|---|---|---|
| 1.0 | 12 | 15 | 0 | 12 | 15 | 0 |

The next set of eight maps (Maps 35–42) documented the work of the PPP staff and partnering agencies in orchestrating the sentencing activities over the two-year period. This was viewed as part of their role as staff and youth serving agencies respectively, and thus did not earn village-building points.

| STORY ID | TEEN COURT | | MAP | 35 | DATE(S) | 10/95 TO 12/95 | |
|---|---|---|---|---|---|---|---|

| WHO | POP | TYPE | DID WHAT | LEVEL | MULT |
|---|---|---|---|---|---|
| STAFF AND AGENCIES | 4 | G | ORCHESTRATED SENTENCING OPTIONS | ACT3 | 0 |

| FOR WHOM | POP | TYPE | WITH WHAT RESULT | LEVEL | MULT |
|---|---|---|---|---|---|
| YOUTH | 24 | C | PARTICIPATED IN SENTENCING OPTIONS | LEV3 | 4 |

| LEVERAGE FRACTION | ACTION POINTS | RECIPIENT POINTS | SELF-DETERMINATION | VILLAGE BUILDING | SERVICES | NETWORKING |
|---|---|---|---|---|---|---|
| 1.0 | 0 | 12 | 0 | 0 | 12 | 0 |

| STORY ID | TEEN COURT | | MAP | 36 | DATE(S) | 1/96 TO 3/96 | |
|---|---|---|---|---|---|---|---|

| WHO | POP | TYPE | DID WHAT | LEVEL | MULT |
|---|---|---|---|---|---|
| STAFF AND AGENCIES | 4 | G | ORCHESTRATED SENTENCING OPTIONS | ACT3 | 0 |

| FOR WHOM | POP | TYPE | WITH WHAT RESULT | LEVEL | MULT |
|---|---|---|---|---|---|
| YOUTH | 24 | C | PARTICIPATED IN SENTENCING OPTIONS | LEV3 | 4 |

| LEVERAGE FRACTION | ACTION POINTS | RECIPIENT POINTS | SELF-DETERMINATION | VILLAGE BUILDING | SERVICES | NETWORKING |
|---|---|---|---|---|---|---|
| 1.0 | 0 | 12 | 0 | 0 | 12 | 0 |

| STORY ID | TEEN COURT | | MAP | 37 | DATE(S) | 4/96 TO 6/96 | |
|---|---|---|---|---|---|---|---|

| WHO | POP | TYPE | DID WHAT | LEVEL | MULT |
|---|---|---|---|---|---|
| STAFF AND AGENCIES | 4 | G | ORCHESTRATED SENTENCING OPTIONS | ACT3 | 0 |

| FOR WHOM | POP | TYPE | WITH WHAT RESULT | LEVEL | MULT |
|---|---|---|---|---|---|
| YOUTH | 30 | C | PARTICIPATED IN SENTENCING OPTIONS | LEV3 | 5 |

| LEVERAGE FRACTION | ACTION POINTS | RECIPIENT POINTS | SELF-DETERMINATION | VILLAGE BUILDING | SERVICES | NETWORKING |
|---|---|---|---|---|---|---|
| 1.0 | 0 | 15 | 0 | 0 | 12 | 0 |

| STORY ID | TEEN COURT | MAP | 38 | DATE(S) | 7/96 TO 9/96 |
|---|---|---|---|---|---|

| WHO | POP | TYPE | DID WHAT | LEVEL | MULT |
|---|---|---|---|---|---|
| STAFF AND AGENCIES | 4 | G | ORCHESTRATED SENTENCING OPTIONS | ACT3 | 0 |

| FOR WHOM | POP | TYPE | WITH WHAT RESULT | LEVEL | MULT |
|---|---|---|---|---|---|
| YOUTH | 30 | C | PARTICIPATED IN SENTENCING OPTIONS | LEV3 | 5 |

| LEVERAGE FRACTION | ACTION POINTS | RECIPIENT POINTS | SELF-DETERMINATION | VILLAGE BUILDING | SERVICES | NETWORKING |
|---|---|---|---|---|---|---|
| 1.0 | 0 | 15 | 0 | 0 | 15 | 0 |

---

| STORY ID | TEEN COURT | MAP | 39 | DATE(S) | 10/96 TO 12/96 |
|---|---|---|---|---|---|

| WHO | POP | TYPE | DID WHAT | LEVEL | MULT |
|---|---|---|---|---|---|
| STAFF AND AGENCIES | 4 | G | ORCHESTRATED SENTENCING OPTIONS | ACT3 | 0 |

| FOR WHOM | POP | TYPE | WITH WHAT RESULT | LEVEL | MULT |
|---|---|---|---|---|---|
| YOUTH | 40 | C | PARTICIPATED IN SENTENCING OPTIONS | LEV3 | 5 |

| LEVERAGE FRACTION | ACTION POINTS | RECIPIENT POINTS | SELF-DETERMINATION | VILLAGE BUILDING | SERVICES | NETWORKING |
|---|---|---|---|---|---|---|
| 1.0 | 0 | 15 | 0 | 0 | 15 | 0 |

---

| STORY ID | TEEN COURT | MAP | 40 | DATE(S) | 1/97 TO 3/97 |
|---|---|---|---|---|---|

| WHO | POP | TYPE | DID WHAT | LEVEL | MULT |
|---|---|---|---|---|---|
| STAFF AND AGENCIES | 4 | G | ORCHESTRATED SENTENCING OPTIONS | ACT3 | 0 |

| FOR WHOM | POP | TYPE | WITH WHAT RESULT | LEVEL | MULT |
|---|---|---|---|---|---|
| YOUTH | 40 | C | PARTICIPATED IN SENTENCING OPTIONS | LEV3 | 5 |

| LEVERAGE FRACTION | ACTION POINTS | RECIPIENT POINTS | SELF-DETERMINATION | VILLAGE BUILDING | SERVICES | NETWORKING |
|---|---|---|---|---|---|---|
| 1.0 | 0 | 15 | 0 | 0 | 15 | 0 |

---

| STORY ID | TEEN COURT | MAP | 41 | DATE(S) | 4/97 TO 6/97 |
|---|---|---|---|---|---|

| WHO | POP | TYPE | DID WHAT | LEVEL | MULT |
|---|---|---|---|---|---|
| STAFF AND AGENCIES | 4 | G | ORCHESTRATED SENTENCING OPTIONS | ACT3 | 0 |

| FOR WHOM | POP | TYPE | WITH WHAT RESULT | LEVEL | MULT |
|---|---|---|---|---|---|
| YOUTH | 30 | C | PARTICIPATED IN SENTENCING OPTIONS | LEV3 | 5 |

| LEVERAGE FRACTION | ACTION POINTS | RECIPIENT POINTS | SELF-DETERMINATION | VILLAGE BUILDING | SERVICES | NETWORKING |
|---|---|---|---|---|---|---|
| 1.0 | 0 | 15 | 0 | 0 | 15 | 0 |

| STORY ID | TEEN COURT | | MAP | 42 | DATE(S) | 7/97 TO 9/97 | |
|---|---|---|---|---|---|---|---|

| WHO | POP | TYPE | DID WHAT | LEVEL | MULT |
|---|---|---|---|---|---|
| STAFF AND AGENCIES | 4 | G | ORCHESTRATED SENTENCING OPTIONS | ACT3 | 0 |

| FOR WHOM | POP | TYPE | WITH WHAT RESULT | LEVEL | MULT |
|---|---|---|---|---|---|
| YOUTH | 22 | C | PARTICIPATED IN SENTENCING OPTIONS | LEV3 | 4 |

| LEVERAGE FRACTION | ACTION POINTS | RECIPIENT POINTS | SELF-DETERMINATION | VILLAGE BUILDING | SERVICES | NETWORKING |
|---|---|---|---|---|---|---|
| 1.0 | 0 | 12 | 0 | 0 | 12 | 0 |

This brings us to the milestones. All of the 240 defendants completed their sentences and only 8 percent (19 of 240) of them were repeat offenders. Recognizing that the youth were sent to Teen Court for relatively minor offenses, and were not "career criminals" with previous records, it was not reasonable to assign a MLS6 code to the outcomes achieved (i.e., there were unlikely to be major lifestyle changes resulting from the Court experience). However, MLS4 codes seemed appropriate, since all 240—including the repeat offenders—engaged in several months of corrective activity (i.e., workshops, jury duty, and writing letters of apology). These intermediate-level milestones were recorded as Maps 43 through 282, one per defendant. Only one of these maps is shown below as an example.

| STORY ID | TEEN COURT | | MAP | 57 | DATE(S) | 10/95 TO 12/95 | |
|---|---|---|---|---|---|---|---|

| WHO | POP | TYPE | DID WHAT | LEVEL | MULT |
|---|---|---|---|---|---|
| YOUTH | 1 | C | TOOK ACTIONS TO DISCOURAGE FUTURE OFFENSES | MLS4 | 1 |

| FOR WHOM | POP | TYPE | WITH WHAT RESULT | LEVEL | MULT |
|---|---|---|---|---|---|
| [SELF] | | | | | |

| LEVERAGE FRACTION | ACTION POINTS | RECIPIENT POINTS | SELF-DETERMINATION | VILLAGE BUILDING | SERVICES | NETWORKING |
|---|---|---|---|---|---|---|
| 1.0 | 4 | 0 | 4 | 0 | 0 | 0 |

The next set of maps (Maps 283–324) is directed at the 42 teen attorneys. By all accounts, this was a major learning experience for them. Several indicated they were now considering careers in law or criminal justice. Again, milestone 4 seemed the appropriate outcome level. Only one map is shown as an example.

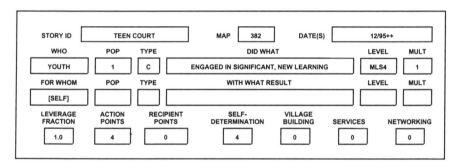

Milestones (MLS4) were also assigned to the 93 youth who served on the juries. They gave up their Saturdays throughout the year to provide this community service for their peers. Many indicated that they gained a lot from their experience and had moderated some of their behaviors. These milestones were documented in Maps 325–417. One such map is shown here as an example.

| STORY ID | TEEN COURT | | MAP | 382 | DATE(S) | | 12/95++ | |
|---|---|---|---|---|---|---|---|---|
| WHO | POP | TYPE | | DID WHAT | | | LEVEL | MULT |
| YOUTH | 1 | C | | ENGAGED IN SIGNIFICANT, NEW LEARNING | | | MLS4 | 1 |
| FOR WHOM | POP | TYPE | | WITH WHAT RESULT | | | LEVEL | MULT |
| [SELF] | | | | | | | | |
| LEVERAGE FRACTION | ACTION POINTS | RECIPIENT POINTS | SELF-DETERMINATION | | VILLAGE BUILDING | SERVICES | | NETWORKING |
| 1.0 | 4 | 0 | 4 | | 0 | 0 | | 0 |

The final set of maps of the story (Maps 418–425) presented the institutional impact. Through the Teen Court experience, a loosely knit coalition strengthened cross-agency ties and has continued to meet and implement projects. While no points were earned for these milestones (since all participants were "doing their job," albeit in a new way), it set the stage for other stories in which the program (PPP) was actively engaged and earned points. One of these maps is provided as an example.

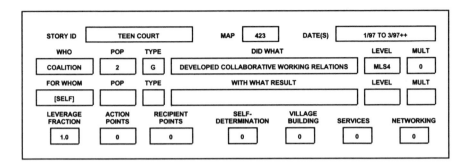

| STORY ID | TEEN COURT | | MAP | 423 | DATE(S) | | 1/97 TO 3/97++ | |
|---|---|---|---|---|---|---|---|---|
| **WHO** | **POP** | **TYPE** | | **DID WHAT** | | | **LEVEL** | **MULT** |
| COALITION | 2 | G | | DEVELOPED COLLABORATIVE WORKING RELATIONS | | | MLS4 | 0 |
| **FOR WHOM** | **POP** | **TYPE** | | **WITH WHAT RESULT** | | | **LEVEL** | **MULT** |
| [SELF] | | | | | | | | |
| **LEVERAGE FRACTION** | **ACTION POINTS** | **RECIPIENT POINTS** | **SELF-DETERMINATION** | **VILLAGE BUILDING** | | **SERVICES** | | **NETWORKING** |
| 1.0 | 0 | 0 | 0 | 0 | | 0 | | 0 |

*Story Summary.* The Teen Court story earned PPP a total of 1701 action points and 543 recipient points. Of the action points, 1,599 points were classified as self-determination (207 for the teen attorneys, 432 for the jury members, and 960 for the defendants) and 102 points as village building (39, 27, and 36 points respectively for the efforts of the adult attorneys, judges, and adults who worked with the parents of the defendants). The 543 service points included 108 cl-I-ent service points directed at the teen attorneys, 30 cl-I-ent service points directed at the jury members, 222 cl-I-ent service points at the defendants, 120 family service points directed at the parents of the defendants, and 15, 27, and 21 volunteer service points directed at the judges, adult attorneys, and adult volunteers respectively.

Staff were the sole change agents in 10 of the 425 maps in the story, in all cases taking actions at results level 3. In addition, they were part of the group activities associated with 16 maps. All other actions (by the judges, teen and adult attorneys, and other youth and adult volunteers) were also at ACT3. The 383 maps with milestones were all at MLS4 and acknowledged the change processes affecting the 240 defendants, 42 teen attorneys, 93 jury members, and the multi-agency coalition.

# QUIZ 7

7.1. Map and score the following story: In January 1997, Ms. Jones, a member of the Hollywood Lutheran Church, began coming to the program's monthly blood pressure screenings. In February, the parish nurse (a program staffer) determined that Ms. Jones' blood pressure had dropped to 80/60. She was immediately referred to Dr. Perry, her physician, who diagnosed her as having a potentially fatal thyroid disorder and provided treatment. Ms. Jones' blood pressure was monitored monthly by the parish nurse (March through June). In May, Ms. Jones—who had not previously performed any community service—volunteered to participate in the program's outreach project for the homebound. During the next two months, she made home visits to 12 homebound church members.

7.2. Map and score Prof. Smith's story: At Central Connecticut University, two program staff recruited five faculty members, including Prof. Smith, in September 1996 who were willing to introduce substance abuse topics within their respective courses. In October, the staff facilitated a series of brainstorming sessions with these five faculty members to determine where best to introduce materials. The five faculty members, working independently, revised their respective courses during the months of November and December. During the next quarter, January through March 1997, 104 students were exposed to the materials in lectures and assignments (23 were Prof. Smith's students). In follow-up interviews with a sample of 26 students in April, including 9 from Prof. Smith's class, staff learned that students were positive about the new content, felt it added realism to the subjects discussed, and thought this type of exposure to issues was far more effective than public service announcements and other warning messages.

7.3. Map and score the following story: Since February 1997, the Caswell Senior Center has offered a clogging program. The instructors are two members of the center who were recruited by the center director and volunteer their time. The center provides space and other assistance, as needed, to the instructors. The Center staff announced the new program through a posted announcement on the center bulletin board and 12 center members signed up. These 12 seniors range in age from 68 to 89. They have been meeting two times each week to practice and have named themselves the Down Home Cloggers. Beginning in August, the group began performing in nursing homes around the county, with residents participating by clapping and tapping their toes. By the end of November 1997, when the story was submitted, they had performed at six homes and brought joy to over 200 persons.

# 8

# Graphing

My dad, Herman Kibel, was an outstanding ten pin bowler. In fact, back in the 1950s on Friday evenings, he would drive from our home in New Jersey across the Hudson River into New York City to participate in the New York Majors. There, at Empire Lanes in Downtown Manhattan, some of the greatest bowlers in the world at that time (Lou Campi, Andy Varipapa, and other bowling hall-of-famers) would compete in team play. As a treat, I would sometimes be allowed to tag along and participate in a magical evening at the lanes—made all the better by the din of balls hitting pins and banter, cigarette and cigar smoke, and the aroma of bitter beer. These experiences did not turn me into a smoker or beer drinker. I did, however, become addicted to scorekeeping.

In those days, there were no electronic scorecards over every lane. Score was kept on sheets at the small table between each pair of lanes. To satisfy the crowds who came to watch the action, large chalkboards were also used to track the progress of games. When it was discovered that I was a whiz at arithmetic, was an accurate pin counter, and could print numbers large and neatly, I was recruited as a chalkboard scorekeeper. What a treat this was for me to mark those X's and \'s.

The bowling scorecard is a simple, yet elegant format for mapping a game. Reading across a completed scorecard, player by player, an individual familiar with the sport can easily re-create the entire game's history. While one cannot tell which, if any, bowler threw left handed, how fast they threw, or which specific pins were knocked down each frame, one can quickly determine how many strikes there were, how many pins were knocked down each frame on both the first and second rolls, how many splits and misses there were, and, of course, what the outcome was (i.e., the final score). And, at a glance, an experienced bowler can catch the whole.

I have been keeping score ever since. I have devised special scorecards for tracking the play of football and basketball games. I even redid the classical baseball scorecard to emphasize the performance of the pitchers rather than the hitters.

It should therefore not be surprising to learn that I have devised a scorecard for graphing stories.

Apart from my lifetime love of scorecards, there was a compelling need for this tool. The mapped stories are often long and difficult to capture as a whole. The points tend to foster analytical thinking—which is good. But I wanted something that would encourage holistic assessment as well. In short, I was looking for a way to grasp immediately how a program contributed toward cl-I-ent milestones across its stories. Did the program's best work have a characteristic signature that set it apart from other programs or other of its own work?

The scorecard in Table 8.1 is now used for this purpose.

To illustrate its use, let me graph Frances' story, which appeared in Chapter 2. That story included these six maps:

Map 1. Frances received warm lunches through the meals-on-wheels program operated by the senior center.

Map 2. The volunteer who delivered the meals (John F.) encouraged her to visit the center after she got well.

Maps 3 and 4. Frances benefitted from services and activities provided by the Center's staff. (Two maps are used following a Results Mapping convention that no map should cover more than a three-month period.)

**Table 8.1.** Results Mapping Summary Scorecard

| Name of program | | | | | | | Story ID | | | |
|---|---|---|---|---|---|---|---|---|---|---|
| 1 | | 2 | | 3 | | ❹ | | 5 | | ❻ | ❼ |
| Direct program interventions | | | | | | | | | | |
| | | | | | | | | | | |
| | | | | | | | | | | |
| | | | | | | | | | | |
| | | | | | | | | | | |
| | | | | | | | | | | |
| Networking with others | | | | | | | | | | |
| | | | | | | | | | | |
| | | | | | | | | | | |
| | | | | | | | | | | |
| | | | | | | | | | | |
| Client contributions to others | | | | | | | | | | |
| | | | | | | | | | | |
| | | | | | | | | | | |

Map 5. Frances attended the center on a regular basis. (This was considered a milestone in her life, as previously she had no contact with individuals her own age in Cincinnati.)

Map 6. She has been volunteering in the kitchen helping to prepare the meals that the program delivers. (This marked an important role change for Frances from that of service recipient to a volunteer engaged in service provision—what we refer to as a "village builder" in Results Mapping.)

The graphed version of the story would appear as shown in Table 8.2:

Each of the maps of the story is placed on a row of the scorecard under the column that matches its results level. Thus, the first map (a transaction between a volunteer staffer and the cl-I-ent at ACT3→LEV3) is placed in the first row, third column; the next map (a transaction at ACT2→LEV2 that is also between the volunteer staffer and the cl-I-ent) is placed in the second row, second column; and so on. Where there are multiple persons involved as change agents or recipients, as in Maps 3 and 4, these are indicated as well.

The cl-I-ent's milestone is placed in the cluster to which it most directly relates. We are not claiming causality (i.e., the services in the cluster did not *cause* the milestone to occur). But we are emphasizing contribution and association of these services with the milestone.

There were no handoffs in this story. The cl-I-ent action to help others (in this case, indirectly, and hence the population count of "0") is graphed in its own cluster at the end of the scorecard.

To close this chapter, scorecards for the three stories mapped in Chapter 7 are offered (as Tables 8.3, 8.4, and 8.5).

**Table 8.2.** Frances' Story Graphed

| Senior center | | | | | | Frances | | | | |
|---|---|---|---|---|---|---|---|---|---|---|
| 1 | | 2 | | 3 | | ❹ | 5 | | ❻ | ❼ |
| Direct program interventions | | | | | | | | | | |
| | | | | VS | C | | | | | |
| | | VS | C | | | | | | | |
| | | | | 2S | C | | | | | |
| | | | | 2S | C | | | | | |
| | | | | | | C | | | | |
| Networking with others | | | | | | | | | | |
| | | | | | | | | | | |
| Client contributions to others | | | | | | | | | | |
| | | | | C | 0X | | | | | |

**Table 8.3.** Fred's Story Graphed

| Montana prevention | | | | | | Fred | | | | |
|---|---|---|---|---|---|---|---|---|---|---|
| 1 | | 2 | | 3 | | ❹ | 5 | | ❻ | ❼ |
| Direct program interventions | | | | | | | | | | |
| | | | | S | C | | | | | |
| | | S | C | | | | | | | |
| | | | | S | C | | | | | |
| | | | | S | C | | | | | |
| | | | | | | C | | | | |
| | | | | | | C | | | | |
| | | | | | | | S | C | | |
| | | | | | | | | | C | |
| | | | | | | | | | C | |
| Networking with others | | | | | | | | | | |
| | | S | P | | | | | | | |
| | | | | P | C | | | | | |
| | | S | P | | | | | | | |
| | | | | VP | C | | | | | |
| | | S | 2X | | | | | | | |
| | | | | VX | C | | | | | |
| | | | | VX | C | | | | | |
| | | | | VX | C | | | | | |
| | | | | VX | C | | | | | |
| Client contributions to others | | | | | | | | | | |
| | | VC | 150X | | | | | | | |

**Table 8.4.** Rick's Story Graphed

| San Jose AIDs project | | | | | | Rick | | | | |
|---|---|---|---|---|---|---|---|---|---|---|
| 1 | | 2 | | 3 | | ❹ | 5 | | ❻ | ❼ |
| Direct program interventions | | | | | | | | | | |
| | | | | S | C | | | | | |
| | | | | S | C | | | | | |
| | | | | S | C | | | | | |
| | | | | S | F | | | | | |
| | | | | S | C | | | | | |
| | | | | S | C | | | | | |
| | | | | S | C | | | | | |
| | | | | | | C | | | | |
| | | | | | | F | | | | |
| | | | | | | | S | C | | |
| | | | | | | | S | F | | |
| | | | | | | | S | C | | |
| | | | | | | | S | F | | |
| | | | | | | | S | C | | |
| | | | | | | | S | F | | |
| | | | | | | | | | C | |
| Networking with others | | | | | | | | | | |
| | | S | G | | | | | | | |
| | | | | G | C | | | | | |
| | | S | G | | | | | | | |
| | | G | F | | | | | | | |
| | | S | G | | | | | | | |
| | | | | G | F | | | | | |
| | | | | G | F | | | | | |
| | | S | G | | | | | | | |
| | | | | G | C | | | | | |
| | | | | G | C | | | | | |
| | | | | | | | VF | C | | |
| | | | | | | | VF | C | | |
| | | | | | | | VF | C | | |

*(continued)*

**Table 8.4.** (*Continued*)

| | | | | | | | | | |
|---|---|---|---|---|---|---|---|---|---|
| Client contributions to others | | | | | | | | | |
| | | VC | 120X | | | | | | |
| | | VC | 120X | | | | | | |
| | | VC | 120X | | | | | | |
| | | VC | 120X | | | | | | |
| | | VC | 120X | | | | | | |

**Table 8.5.** Pima Teen Court Story Graphed

| Pima prevention | | | | Teen Court | | | |
|---|---|---|---|---|---|---|---|
| 1 | 2 | 3 | ❹ | 5 | ❻ | ❼ | |
| Direct program interventions | | | | | | | |
| | | 2S | 20C | | | | |
| | | 2S | 50C | | | | |
| | | 2S | 22C | | | | |
| | | 2S | 43C | | | | |
| | | 2G | 24C | | | | |
| | | 2G | 24C | | | | |
| | | 2G | 30C | | | | |
| | | 2G | 30C | | | | |
| | | 2G | 40C | | | | |
| | | 2G | 40C | | | | |
| | | 2G | 30C | | | | |
| | | 2G | 22C | | | | |
| | | | 240C | | | | |
| | | | 42C | | | | |
| | | | 93C | | | | |
| | | | 2G | | | | |

**Table 8.5.** (*Continued*)

| | | | | | | | | | | |
|---|---|---|---|---|---|---|---|---|---|---|
| Networking with others | | | | | | | | | | |
| | | | | 2S | 7P | | | | | |
| | | | | 8VP | 10C | | | | | |
| | | | | 9VP | 10C | | | | | |
| | | | | 7VP | 10C | | | | | |
| | | | | 12VP | 15C | | | | | |
| | | | | 2S | 30P | | | | | |
| | | | | 4VP | 24C | | | | | |
| | | | | 4VP | 24C | | | | | |
| | | | | 6VP | 30C | | | | | |
| | | | | 5VP | 30C | | | | | |
| | | | | 2S | 18X | | | | | |
| | | | | 6VX | 40F | | | | | |
| | | | | 8VX | 40F | | | | | |
| | | | | 8VX | 40F | | | | | |
| | | | | 10VX | 40F | | | | | |
| | | | | 2S | 2P | | | | | |
| | | | | 12VP | 15C | | | | | |
| | | | | 14VP | 13C | | | | | |
| | | | | 11VP | 15C | | | | | |
| | | | | 7VP | 10C | | | | | |
| | | | | 2S | 15P | | | | | |
| | | | | 6VP | 40C | | | | | |
| | | | | 7VP | 40C | | | | | |
| | | | | 8VP | 30C | | | | | |
| | | | | 6VP | 22C | | | | | |
| | | | | 2S | 9X | | | | | |
| | | | | 11VX | 40F | | | | | |
| | | | | 15VX | 40F | | | | | |
| | | | | 15VX | 40F | | | | | |
| | | | | 11VX | 40F | | | | | |

(*continued*)

**Table 8.5.** (*Continued*)

| | | | | Client contributions to others | | | | | | |
|---|---|---|---|---|---|---|---|---|---|---|
| | | | | 10C | — | | | | | |
| | | | | 26C | — | | | | | |
| | | | | 10C | — | | | | | |
| | | | | 29C | — | | | | | |
| | | | | 10C | — | | | | | |
| | | | | 32C | — | | | | | |
| | | | | 15C | — | | | | | |
| | | | | 40C | — | | | | | |
| | | | | 15C | — | | | | | |
| | | | | 53C | — | | | | | |
| | | | | 13C | — | | | | | |
| | | | | 51C | — | | | | | |
| | | | | 15C | — | | | | | |
| | | | | 42C | — | | | | | |
| | | | | 10C | — | | | | | |
| | | | | 38C | — | | | | | |

# Glossary of Key Terms

**Action points**    Points earned by the program for actions initiated by volunteers or by the program's cl-I-ents and their families.

**Assisted handoff**    A handoff sequence in which the cl-I-ent takes unusual action or is helped to follow-through with the new change agent who has received the handoff.

**Change agent**    The person(s) or entity initiating an action that is mapped.

**Cl-I-ents**    The individuals, families, teams, organizations, neighborhoods, communities, or systems that are featured in a program's top stories. The capital "I" reminds us of the program's challenge to help its cl-I-ents reach the stage at which they take responsibility for their own growth and health.

**Handoff**    A map documenting the transfer of responsibility for the next action to another change agent. Always coded as ACT2→LEV2.

**Hard data**    Data that are accurate, have face validity, and are consistent with the best current science from any fields in which the latest truths and insights are being generated.

**Map**    The basic unit and building block of a story that describes in structured format the actions taken by a change agent(s) to benefit self or others, as well as the benefits—if any—that accrue to a recipient(s). Also referred to as a mapping sentence.

**Map leverage fraction**    A fraction with values of 1.0, 0.5, or 0.0 used in computing action and recipient points. The fraction is used to discount a program's points when (1) the change agent has not been in direct contact with the program or (2) the results level achieved is two or more levels higher than the highest level of related staff action in the story.

**Map score**    The sum of the action points and recipient points earned by the program for one map.

**Milestone**    Rung 4, 6, or 7 of the Results Ladder and the corresponding advance in status of a cl-I-ent, a family member, or a community group. Akin to an "outcome."

141

**Networking points**   Recipient points earned by the program when a hand-off is made to another service provider.

**Program**   The entity that is being evaluated.

**Population multiplier**   A multiplier with integer values ranging from 0 to 10 used in computing action and recipient points. The multiplier is a quasi-logarithmic conversion of the number of change agents or recipients in a map. The multiplier may be assigned values of 0 or 1 in lieu of the converted value to account for specific situations and role types.

**Recipient**   The person(s) or entity featured in a map who is affected by, or received the benefit of the actions of a change agent(s).

**Recipient points**   Points earned by the program for services received by recipients (e.g., by cl-I-ents or other family or community members) or for networking with another provider.

**Results ladder**   A seven-stage framework used for coding effects on, and changes in the status of, cl-I-ents and other community members included in a story.

**Results level**   A rung of the Results Ladder. Used to refer to the numeric position of an action or benefit on the Ladder.

**Self-determination points**   Action points earned for self-referential maps (i.e., for actions taken for self or for future benefit of others).

**Self-referential map**   A map with a change agent(s) but no recipient. The benefit is for the change agent(s) or some future recipient(s).

**Service points**   Recipient points earned by the program for benefits received by recipients (other than for networking).

**Split map**   A transactional map that is presented as multiple maps to account for different types of change agents or recipients.

**Story**   A set of maps organized in roughly chronological order that describes the actions taken by program staff and by others that the staff have mobilized (including the cl-I-ent) to influence the health and growth of the cl-I-ent featured in the story.

**Story score**   The sum of all map scores in the story.

**Transactional map**   A map with both change agent(s) and recipient(s).

**Type code**   A letter code used to designate the type of change agent(s) or recipient(s) of a map.

**Village-building points**   Action points earned for transactional maps when the change agent is a volunteer.

# Appendix A

## Answers to the Quizzes

*1.1. As commonly used, what are the differences between program inputs, outputs, outcomes, impacts, and results?*

Program *inputs* refer to the labor and other resources that go into providing program services (e.g., staff hours, volunteer hours, equipment, facilities). Program *outputs* refer to the immediate effects of these services expressed in output units (e.g., 10 youth trained, 12 home visits to new parents, 35 blood pressure screenings provided). *Outcomes* refer to positive behavior or status changes linked to these outputs (e.g., stopped smoking, agreed to participate in family therapy, maintained new diet for six months, graduated from high school). These are reflective of the goals of the program and may be interim (i.e., short-lived), short-term (i.e., the effects lasting at least one month following the interventions), or sustained for longer time periods. Impacts carry two widely different meanings, depending on the discipline using the term. *Impacts* are sometimes used to refer to interim outcomes (i.e., the immediate outcomes stemming from services provided), but at other times used to refer to systemic or community-wide outcomes expressed as social or community indicators (e.g., reduction in city-wide drug use, higher rates of employment, or lower alcohol-linked traffic fatalities). *Results* are most generic and include all of the above except inputs.

*1.2. When does it make sense to invest evaluation dollars in outcome measurement? When does it make sense to invest evaluation dollars in community impact measurement? And when would it make more sense to invest these dollars in an approach such as Results Mapping?*

*Outcome measurement* is ideally suited for relatively closed systems evaluations, where interventions are standardized, clients are similar, outside influences can be controlled, and one or a few clearly defined and measurable outcomes are being targeted. For example, the value of a program that provides free flu shots each fall at schools and workplaces could be fairly determined through outcome measurement. Similarly, an after-school program aimed at building resiliency in the youth participants could be assessed in terms of this challenge (e.g., using a pre–post instrument that gauges resiliency levels). Investments in *community impact measurement* make sense when a single or a few interrelated interventions are being directed at all or a large segment of the overall community population, where the interventions are logically connected to the impacts desired, and other factors and forces influencing these impacts in the same direction can be demonstrated to be less significant than the interventions. For example, the consequences of a state-level policy to reduce the legal drinking age from 21 to 19 could be determined with reasonable accuracy through an impact study. In most other cases, *Results Mapping or a similar approach that bridges program actions to outcomes* is likely to add most value for the evaluation dollar. In some situations, a blended approach may be most beneficial (e.g., combining outcome measurement addressing short-term outcomes with Results Mapping to bridge to the longer-term outcomes).

*1.3. What makes prevention programs more difficult to evaluate than treatment programs? What is the "bottom line" against which prevention programs ought to be judged?*

Prevention programs aim at outcomes that are beyond the period of direct influence of the program and also likely to be beyond the time frame of the evaluation. The "bottom line" for prevention programs is the extent of contribution they make toward lowering the probabilities of unwanted future outcomes and raising the probabilities of desired future outcomes. The "bottom line" for a treatment program is a cured person (or, at least, one less likely to relapse). It is easier to count cured persons than to assign probabilities to future behaviors and status. Unless treatment programs have "magic bullets" to offer their clients, they may be well advised to adopt prevention's bottom line.

*2.1. Why does Results Mapping focus on a program's* best *stories? Wouldn't we get more reliable information regarding the overall program by random sampling? Also, shouldn't a program's worse stories be studied to discover what the program is doing wrong and needs to correct?*

As long as effective work in promoting client growth and transformation is relatively rare, it is only the program's top 10–20 stories that will reveal much program success in this area. Most of the program's remaining stories will consist solely of short-term services provided and immediate benefits received. Through random sampling, we would get only a few "hits" with stories featuring any type of growth and thus have little material to learn from. By concentrating at the top end, we draw on all or most of the stories from which learning can occur.

A program's worse stories, in a Results Mapping sense, are those with few maps and low scores. There is no material here to use for learning. However, where the intent is to correct program deficiencies that lead to unsatisfied or under-served clients, a different type of evaluation (or applying Results Mapping to a subset of clients who are not performing well—for example, to the "best stories" of boys with attention deficits) makes more sense than looking only at the pro-gram's top stories.

*2.2. Why do total quality management principles (e.g., working for zero defects, visible measures of performance, and shared responsibility for quality out-put) work better when applied to factory production systems than to social service or prevention programs?*

In factory-like systems (e.g., an appliance manufacturer or a fast food fran-chise), there is a standard, perfect product (or products) that the system needs to replicate—and can replicate—again and again. Any deviation from the perfect product is a cause for concern and action. The challenge is to minimize cross-item differences, with *zero difference* being the ultimate mark of success. In social ser-vice or prevention systems, particularly the types best suited for study through Re-sults Mapping, the challenge is to maximize client health and growth. The mark of success is *maximum positive change, client by client*, from the statuses at which the program begins to interact with them. Although such programs work for the mirror opposite of zero defects, they can benefit from applications of other total quality management principles, such as visible measures of performance (albeit more difficult to measure than hamburger circumference) and shared responsibil-ity for quality output (via program use of learning communities and group prob-lem-solving sessions).

*2.3. Is it possible to be "objective" when the unit of analysis is a story? Are num-bers inherently more objective than stories?*

A number is more objective than a story because it is more object-like—it is singular and static, whereas a story has multiple aspects and flows. However, ob-jectivity can be an over-rated criterion. One can be objective about "objects" but far less so about people and human systems. In fact, even for objects, there is a lot of ambiguity if one digs deep enough. Behaviors at subatomic levels appear to de-pend on the experimental situation (i.e., the electron will act like a particle or like a wave, depending on the type of apparatus the scientist is causing it to interact with) and not on any fixed truth. A better criterion for rating numbers versus stories is *fi-delity*, namely how well each reflects and captures the richness of the reality being represented. When mapped correctly, stories always have more fidelity than numbers alone have. All this having been said, complete narrative accounts do lead to consistent ratings from independent coders and scorers and thereby meet certain standards of "objectivity" as commonly understood.

*3.1. Johnny viewed a public service announcement on television that warned against the use of chewing tobacco. What level did this represent for him?*

     Johnny reached LEV1. He indirectly received information of general nature.

*3.2. The team put up anti-drug posters around the school. What was this action level?*

     The team functioned at ACT1. They distributed information of general nature to all students at the school (LEV1). If, prior to the distribution, they were trained in producing posters, this would be a LEV3 service provided to them—but not to the other students at the school.

*3.3. Dave, a recovering alcoholic, established a support group for co-workers from his office that meets weekly. Dave reported having reached his first anniversary without a drink. What was the personal milestone level reached by Dave? When can support group members begin receiving milestones for their accomplishments? At what milestone level?*

     Dave personally reached MLS6 (more than six months with a sustained, positive behavior). Milestones (MLS4s) can be claimed for support group members after a month of participation and sustained changes in their drinking behaviors. Their participation in the group is coded at ACT3→LEV3 for the first six months and, if these milestones are reached, at ACT5→LEV5 thereafter. Like Dave, they can achieve MLS6s after more than six months of sustained behavior and associated lifestyle changes.

*3.4. Dr. Smith suggested that Sally call the child care center to seek placement for her child. At what action level was Dr. Smith operating? What was the benefit level for Sally?*

     The doctor was operating at ACT2 and Sally was benefitting at LEV2. Should she follow through on the referral, higher levels might be reached for her and her child.

*3.5. Marie, who had not been following her doctor's advice regarding her diet, almost died. Following an emergency intervetnion, she began monitoring her diet closely and has not had a recurring medical problem in nine months.* What levels has she been operating at during these nine months and what personal milestones has she reached?

In maintaining a new diet for nine months, Marie would have been mapped twice at ACT3 (for self-benefit) and once at ACT5 (again for self-benefit). She would also have been assigned a MLS4 after the first month for sticking to the diet after ignoring her doctor's earlier advice. By month 9, Marie has reached MLS6. She has made a sustained adjustment in her lifestyle in the direction of improved health.

*3.6. Jennie is a fantastic trainer. She conducted a three-hour workshop for 15 trainees. Larry, a boring trainer, conducted the same three-hour workshop for 15 different trainees. At what action level was Jennie operating? At what action level was Larry operating?*

Both Jennie and Larry were operating at ACT3. The quality of services is not reflected in the determination of change agent level. The quality issue is reflected in the total story score, not in any single map score. If Jennie is truly a better trainer, then her stories will score higher when trainees follow through on the skills and options transferred to them.

*3.7. Frank agreed to serve as a mentor for young Arnie. For a year, he met with Arnie three times a week to help with reading and homework and to take Arnie on outings to museums and sporting events. Arnie often initiates calls to Frank for advice and is now talking about becoming a mentor for a younger child.* What level of relationship developed between Frank and Arnie by the end of the year? Is there any indication of a milestone for Arnie and, if so, at what level?

Their relationship at year end was at ACT5→LEV5. There were multiple services, two-way interaction, and the shifting of the locus of control from Frank to Arnie. From the limited information provided, it does seem that Arnie has made some adjustments in his behaviors that warrant a MLS4. If he actually becomes a mentor and maintains this relationship for more than six months, it should warrant a MLS6 as well.

*3.8. Maurice suffers from Alzheimer's disease. He has attended an adult day center daily for the past eight months, where he spends his day being a passive recipient of services. Thanks to the center, his daughter, who is Maurice's primary care giver, has been able to keep her job and get some respite.* What is the highest milestone Maurice can reach? What milestone has his daughter reached?

This is a tricky example. The goal is to keep Maurice out of an expensive and possibly impersonal nursing home for as long as feasible. By attending the day center, Maurice has benefitted at LEV3 (i.e., he has received meals, stimulation, and attention). However, due to his disease and lack of short-term memory, he cannot advance to MLS4 (i.e., he cannot initiate and sustain actions to change his status). Although the service is offered daily, it cannot be coded as ACT5→LEV5, since the locus of control cannot shift to Maurice. His daughter is also benefitting from the LEV3 services to her father through the respite provided. Additionally, a MLS4 can be credited for her adjustments to accommodate the routine of work and day care for her father. A MLS6 would not be warranted. It is too far removed (i.e., three levels) from the type of benefits she is getting from the day center.

*3.9. On the July 4th weekend, the local police were out in force checking for intoxicated drivers.* At what level were they operating? Who were their "clients"?

This is another tricky example. The police were engaged in a routine ACT2→LEV2 interaction with drivers stopped who were not intoxicated, as well as with other drivers or would-be drivers from the community who were made aware of the roadside checks. However, for those drivers who were stopped and found to be intoxicated (i.e., their blood alcohol concentration levels were above the legal limit), the service was likely extended beyond motivation to an ACT3→LEV3 interchange (albeit not a happy one for the drivers). Two maps would be needed to capture the two types of exchanges—with the drivers in each category (i.e., those impacted at LEV2 and at LEV3) being the recipients of the two maps respectively.

The community at large could also be considered as indirect recipients of the police actions—since the roads were safer. However, this would typically not be mapped. More typically, an impact type of evaluation would be used rather than Results Mapping to document and measure this broad level of community impact.

*4.1. When would a story be split into two or more separate stories?*

A story is split into two or more separate stories whenever the featured cl-I-ent changes. For example, a story that begins with a youth may spin off into a second story involving his sister who has subsequently become a cl-I-ent and made major gains of her own. If these gains had been modest, she would have been treated and mapped as a family member in her brother's story. When splitting a story, it is acceptable to have some of the same maps appearing in both stories. This "double counting" is unlikely to be significant enough to influence the findings or recommendations from the story data.

*4.2. What change agent type (S or VS) would be assigned to a teenager who worked for the program during the summer and was paid minimum wage?*

Minimum wage is considered a fair wage for a day's work. Therefore, the teenager would not be considered a volunteer and would be coded as staff ("S"). As explained in Chapter 6, this means that the program would not earn village building points for actions initiated by the student.

*4.3. What change agent type (S or VS) would be assigned to a teenager who worked for the program for two months to satisfy her school's community service requirement?*

Although the student is required to do community service, she is still doing this as a volunteer. Hence, she would be coded as "VS" and, as explained in Chapter 6, could earn village-building points for the program.

*4.4. How many maps would be included in a story to show that a cl-I-ent attended weekly support group meetings for four months?*

There would be two maps, the first covering the initial three months of participation and the second map covering the fourth month (according to our convention for repeated services).

*4.5. A program's best story dated back to 1993, but is ongoing (i.e., services are still being provided to the featured cl-I-ent). When it maps that story and computes its score, is it possible that the story will not score very high? If so, is something wrong with the scoring system?*

In most cases, if the story is ongoing, we would expect to see the cl-I-ent now operating at LEV5 and providing assistance to other cl-I-ents or community members. Hence, the story would still score reasonably high even when only the last two years of maps are scored. If the scores are low, this suggests that the cl-I-ent has relapsed and is now receiving only a few basic services or that recent contact with the program, while ongoing, is sporadic. There is nothing wrong here with the scoring system.

*5.1. What are likely causes of staff frustration or concern when they first start capturing their top stories using Results Mapping? What might be done to reduce or eliminate these?*

A first reaction is that this seems like more work for the staff. Further, they have to learn a new vocabulary and mapping rules and convention. It has to be explained to them that all beginnings seem difficult, but once they get used to mapping stories, the extra time required is not excessive and is warranted given the chance to showcase their best work—perhaps for the first time. A second concern is that the quality of the stories themselves is usually lower than expected, particularly if a program has not engaged in follow-up activities with its cl-I-ents. Staff need to recognize that Results Mapping represents a shift in philosophy toward the cl-I-ent-as-resource model and that the program may have been encouraged by its funders and others to be a lower-scoring, service-centered model until now. So it's not their fault that the stories are relatively low-scoring. Third, despite the new philosophy, they may feel that they are still expected to deliver services and not engage much, if at all, in less direct and tangible activities. The program leadership and particularly funders must assure them that these latter types of activities are what is now expected.

*5.2. What program actions are most likely to lead to increases in points during the first months of using Results Mapping? What actions are most likely to lead to these increases after five to six months? What about after a year?*

During the initial months, dramatic point gains occur when staff re-map their stories based on feedback provided by us or other experienced mappers. They recognize that they have failed to take enough credit for all the direct and leveraged activities they have promoted. At the half-year mark, most gains in points result from better story documentation. Programs have taken the time to talk to cl-I-ents or other providers and learn of progress for which they deserve full or partial credit. After a year, most gains in points are derived from new program activities of the types that the point system favors, namely those that promote networking, village building, and cl-I-ent empowerment.

*5.3. What arguments would you use to gain support for Results Mapping from a key stakeholder (funder or political leader) who feels pressured to show that funds being spent are making a real difference in the community?*

One might argue that (1) significant shifts in community indicators take time and large resource commitments, and are hard to link to any specific program activity, (2) stories reveal more about a program's real contributions to these shifts than do numbers, (3) Results Mapping allows stories to be quantified and used as a basis for both ongoing assessment and continual program improvement, and (4) data from mapped stories are as "hard" (i.e., as high in utility and fidelity) as one can get to measure the work of programs engaged in healing, transformation, and prevention.

*6.1. How is progress different on a developmental hierarchy (stage-to-stage development) than on the Results Ladder?*

While slippage is possible, movement on a developmental hierarchy is in one continuous direction and usually tied to ages and stages of life. Movement on the Results Ladder also points upward (i.e., toward MLS6 and MLS7), but the maps may include activities at varying results levels depending on the services provided and the responses to these. Further, a cl-I-ent may be pursuing multiple longer-term outcomes and be at different positions on the Ladder with regard to each such outcome.

*6.2. What is the dilemma facing staff-driven programs when it comes to scoring more points based on Results Mapping? What is the way out of this dilemma?*

There is only so much staff can do. If they are providing services, they cannot be using that time and energy to network with other providers or to mobilize volunteers to support their work. If all or most cl-I-ent services are provided by staff, there will be a ceiling effect: they will peak as a program prior to realizing their full potential. This will also show up in their Results Mapping scores, since there will be few, if any, networking and village building points. To grow as a program beyond that ceiling, the program must transform. This means re-inventing the roles of staff as agents of both program and cl-I-ent growth rather than merely as service providers.

*6.3. Why should a program be interested in increasing the percentage of story points earned that are associated with non-staff actions?*

It takes a whole village to raise a child. By extension, it takes a whole community to promote the growth and health of its members. The increase in percentage of points associated with non-staff actions suggests that the program is contributing to the village building process.

*6.4. If a program is a short-term service provider, but also networks with other agencies that engage in longer-term interactions with cl-I-ents, can the program ever earn points when one of its cl-I-ents achieves a long-term milestone (i.e., MLS6 or MLS7)?*

No, it cannot. As a short-term service provider, a program's highest level of activity will be ACT3→LEV3. In networking, it will be functioning at results level

. 2. When its cl-I-ents achieve milestones at levels 6 or 7, these milestones are too many results levels above direct program actions to earn the program any credit for them. At best, the program can get full credit when a cl-I-ent achieves MLS4 and half credit for activities generated by other providers at ACT5→LEV5.

*6.5. Can a program ever earn full credit for a self-referential map coded as MLS7?*

No, it cannot. The highest level of program action possible is ACT5→LEV5. Should a cl-I-ent reach MLS7, this would be two levels higher and result in a map leverage fraction of 0.5. Thus, MLS7 serves as an ideal, but not as an achievable program target for which the program can take full credit (at least for scoring purposes).

*7.1. This is how I mapped and scored the parish nurse story:*

*Maps 1 and 2.* Ms. Jones obtained blood pressure screenings from the parish nurse for the period from January through June (a brief service rather than informative, hence coded at Level 3). Since this covered a six-month period, two maps were needed. These might have been included as Maps 1 and 4 to maintain a strict chronological order, but it is easier to map a repeated service all at once. Further, if Map 1 only covered January and February, then two maps would have been needed later to cover the March through June period—and this would be modest over-counting of points for the services received. Since the parish nurse was program staff (and there was no indication that the nurse was a volunteer), there were no action (and village building) points associated with these two maps. In each map, there were 3 client service points (i.e., Level 3 for 1 person).

| STORY ID | MS. JONES | | MAP | 1 | DATE(S) | | 1/97 TO 3/97 |
|---|---|---|---|---|---|---|---|

| WHO | POP | TYPE | DID WHAT | | LEVEL | MULT |
|---|---|---|---|---|---|---|
| PARISH NURSE | 1 | S | PROVIDED BLOOD PRESSURE SCREENING | | ACT3 | 0 |

| FOR WHOM | POP | TYPE | WITH WHAT RESULT | | LEVEL | MULT |
|---|---|---|---|---|---|---|
| MS. JONES | 1 | C | GOT INDICATION OF HER HEALTH STATUS | | LEV3 | 1 |

| LEVERAGE FRACTION | ACTION POINTS | RECIPIENT POINTS | SELF-DETERMINATION | VILLAGE BUILDING | SERVICES | NETWORKING |
|---|---|---|---|---|---|---|
| 1.0 | 0 | 3 | 0 | 0 | 3 | 0 |

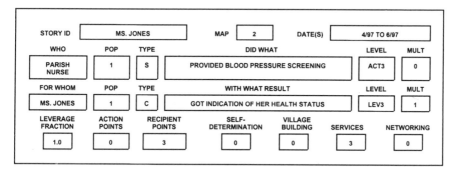

*Maps 3 and 4.* This pair of maps covered the handoff from the parish nurse to the doctor and the subsequent services provided by the latter. By convention, handoffs are coded at Level 2 and the recipient population is 1. This led to 2 recipient points in Map 3, which were classified as networking points. Again, no action points were earned in Map 3, since the change agent was a paid staffer.

The service provided by the doctor in Map 4 was at Level 3. Since the doctor was presumably paid for the services, he was not categorized as a volunteer. Hence, there were no action (and village building) points earned in Map 4, but there were 3 client service points. The leverage fraction remained 1.0, since Dr. Perry was only one step removed from the staff (via the handoff in Map 3).

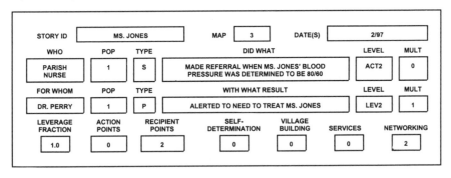

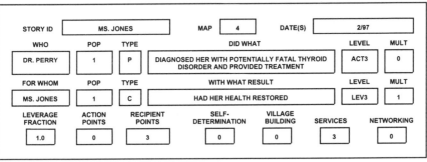

*Maps 5 and 6.* The last two maps in the story featured Ms. Jones in her volunteer role. Map 5 presented her home visits, during a two-month period, to 12 homebound church members. The 12 recipients carry a population multiplier of 4, leading to 12 recipient (and service) points to congregation members (coded as X). Here, action (and village points) were earned since Ms. Jones was a volunteer (and coded as VC to emphasize this). The leverage fraction was 1.0 because Ms. Jones was only one step separated from the staff *and* the Level 3 activity was the same as the earlier Level 3 interaction with staff.

A MLS4 was awarded in Map 6 to document her moving into a new mode of behavior (i.e., community service) and maintaining this new role for more than one month. This earned 4 action points that were classified as self-determination points. The leverage fraction was also 1.0 because Ms. Jones was only one step separated from the staff *and* the Level 4 milestone was only one step higher than the earlier Level 3 interaction with staff.

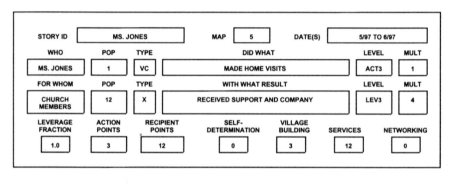

*7.2. This is how I mapped and scored Prof. Smith's story:*

*Map 1.* Two program staff recruited five faculty members in September 1996 for the project (ACT2→LEV2). Recruitment is always considered a Level 2 activity (i.e., motivational). Among the recruits was Prof. Smith. Since it is *his* story being mapped, the number of recipients in Map 1 is shown as 1 and not as 5. Thus, this map earned 2 client service points (2 × 1 = 2). There were no action points, since the change agents were staff.

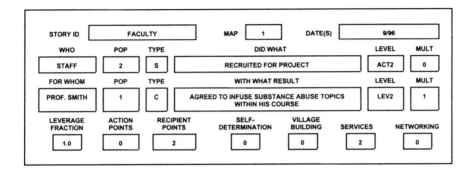

*Map 2.* In October, the staff facilitated a series of brainstorming sessions with these five faculty members (ACT3→LEV3). Again the focus is on Prof. Smith and not on the four others, leading to 3 client service points. And again, there were no action points.

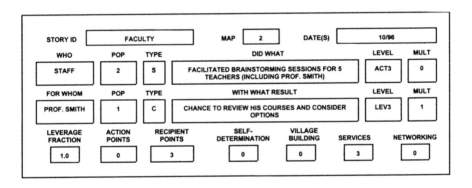

*Map 3.* Prof. Smith, independently of his four colleagues, revised his course during the months of November and December. This was mapped as an ACT3 activity for "future benefit" to students. This was considered an act of self-determination for Prof. Smith. The leverage fraction applied was 1.0, since he was one step removed from staff who had previously interacted with him at Level 3, the same level as this map.

| STORY ID | FACULTY | | | MAP | 3 | DATE(S) | | 11/96 TO 12/96 |
|---|---|---|---|---|---|---|---|---|
| **WHO** | **POP** | **TYPE** | | **DID WHAT** | | | **LEVEL** | **MULT** |
| PROF. SMITH | 1 | C | | MADE REVISIONS TO ONE OF HIS COURSES | | | ACT3 | 1 |
| **FOR WHOM** | **POP** | **TYPE** | | **WITH WHAT RESULT** | | | **LEVEL** | **MULT** |
| [FUTURE] | | | | | | | | |

| LEVERAGE FRACTION | ACTION POINTS | RECIPIENT POINTS | SELF-DETERMINATION | VILLAGE BUILDING | SERVICES | NETWORKING |
|---|---|---|---|---|---|---|
| 1.0 | 3 | 0 | 3 | 0 | 0 | 0 |

*Map 4.* During the next quarter, January through March 1997, 23 of Prof. Smith's students were exposed to the materials in lectures and assignments (ACT3→LEV3). The population multiplier for the services received by the 23 students was 4, leading to 12 service points (3 × 4 = 12). Prof. Smith was considered a village builder. Although he was paid to teach, this additional effort on his part was done on a volunteer basis and involved extra effort. Thus, the map earned an additional 3 × 1 = 3 village-building points. The leverage fraction was 1.0 following the same logic as applied in Map 3.

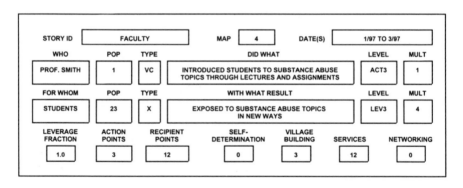

| STORY ID | FACULTY | | | MAP | 4 | DATE(S) | | 1/97 TO 3/97 |
|---|---|---|---|---|---|---|---|---|
| **WHO** | **POP** | **TYPE** | | **DID WHAT** | | | **LEVEL** | **MULT** |
| PROF. SMITH | 1 | VC | | INTRODUCED STUDENTS TO SUBSTANCE ABUSE TOPICS THROUGH LECTURES AND ASSIGNMENTS | | | ACT3 | 1 |
| **FOR WHOM** | **POP** | **TYPE** | | **WITH WHAT RESULT** | | | **LEVEL** | **MULT** |
| STUDENTS | 23 | X | | EXPOSED TO SUBSTANCE ABUSE TOPICS IN NEW WAYS | | | LEV3 | 4 |
| **LEVERAGE FRACTION** | **ACTION POINTS** | **RECIPIENT POINTS** | **SELF-DETERMINATION** | **VILLAGE BUILDING** | **SERVICES** | **NETWORKING** |
| 1.0 | 3 | 12 | 0 | 3 | 12 | 0 |

*Map 5.* A milestone (MLS4) was awarded to Prof. Smith for a new mode of behavior. The leverage fraction was 1.0, since he is one step removed from the program staff who provided service to him (Map 2) and that service (LEV 3) was only one step lower than the milestone level claimed in the map.

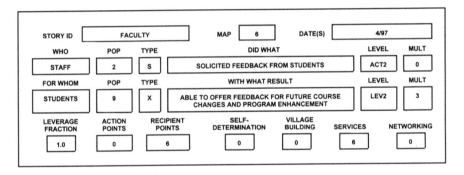

| STORY ID | FACULTY | | MAP | 5 | DATE(S) | | 1/97 TO 3/97 |
|---|---|---|---|---|---|---|---|
| WHO | POP | TYPE | | DID WHAT | | LEVEL | MULT |
| PROF. SMITH | 1 | C | | ADAPTED A NEW APPROACH FOR COMBINING HIS TEACHING WITH SOCIAL RESPONSIBILITY | | MLS4 | 1 |
| FOR WHOM | POP | TYPE | | WITH WHAT RESULT | | LEVEL | MULT |
| [SELF] | | | | | | | |
| LEVERAGE FRACTION | ACTION POINTS | RECIPIENT POINTS | SELF-DETERMINATION | VILLAGE BUILDING | SERVICES | NETWORKING | |
| 1.0 | 4 | 0 | 4 | 0 | 0 | 0 | |

*Map 6.* In follow-up interviews with a sample of 26 students (9 from Prof. Smith's class) in April, staff solicited feedback (ACT2→LEV2). As change agents, the staff do not earn action points. However, there were 2 × 3 = 6 service points (for giving the nine students a chance to express their views).

| STORY ID | FACULTY | | MAP | 6 | DATE(S) | | 4/97 |
|---|---|---|---|---|---|---|---|
| WHO | POP | TYPE | | DID WHAT | | LEVEL | MULT |
| STAFF | 2 | S | | SOLICITED FEEDBACK FROM STUDENTS | | ACT2 | 0 |
| FOR WHOM | POP | TYPE | | WITH WHAT RESULT | | LEVEL | MULT |
| STUDENTS | 9 | X | | ABLE TO OFFER FEEDBACK FOR FUTURE COURSE CHANGES AND PROGRAM ENHANCEMENT | | LEV2 | 3 |
| LEVERAGE FRACTION | ACTION POINTS | RECIPIENT POINTS | SELF-DETERMINATION | VILLAGE BUILDING | SERVICES | NETWORKING | |
| 1.0 | 0 | 6 | 0 | 0 | 6 | 0 | |

*7.3. This is how I mapped and scored the cloggers' story:*

*Maps 1–5.* The instructors were recruited by the center director, then supported with class space and other logistics over a 10-month period. The first map was coded as a recruitment activity, ACT→LEV2. The next four maps (one per three-month period) were coded as ACT3→LEV3, since these were ongoing services provided to the two by the staff (but far short of coaching or mentoring). In all five maps, there were no action points (staff were the change agents). There were 2 × 2 = 4 recipient points in Map 1 and 3 × 2 = 6 recipient points in Maps 2–5. Throughout the story, the two instructors were coded as C for clients (as members of the center), while viewed as volunteer staff.

| STORY ID | CLOGGERS | | MAP | 1 | | DATE(S) | | 2/97 |
|----------|----------|--|-----|---|--|---------|--|------|

| WHO | POP | TYPE | DID WHAT | LEVEL | MULT |
|-----|-----|------|----------|-------|------|
| DIRECTOR | 1 | S | RECRUITED MEMBERS TO TEACH CLOGGING | ACT2 | 0 |

| FOR WHOM | POP | TYPE | WITH WHAT RESULT | LEVEL | MULT |
|----------|-----|------|------------------|-------|------|
| INSTRUCTORS | 2 | C | ENABLED TO TEACH CLOGGING CLASS | LEV2 | 2 |

| LEVERAGE FRACTION | ACTION POINTS | RECIPIENT POINTS | SELF-DETERMINATION | VILLAGE BUILDING | SERVICES | NETWORKING |
|-------------------|---------------|------------------|--------------------|------------------|----------|------------|
| 1.0 | 0 | 4 | 0 | 0 | 4 | 0 |

| STORY ID | CLOGGERS | | MAP | 2 | | DATE(S) | | 2/97 TO 4/97 |
|----------|----------|--|-----|---|--|---------|--|--------------|

| WHO | POP | TYPE | DID WHAT | LEVEL | MULT |
|-----|-----|------|----------|-------|------|
| DIRECTOR | 1 | S | SUPPORTED CLOGGING PROGRAM WITH RESOURCES | ACT3 | 0 |

| FOR WHOM | POP | TYPE | WITH WHAT RESULT | LEVEL | MULT |
|----------|-----|------|------------------|-------|------|
| INSTRUCTORS | 2 | C | ENABLED TO TEACH CLOGGING CLASS | LEV3 | 2 |

| LEVERAGE FRACTION | ACTION POINTS | RECIPIENT POINTS | SELF-DETERMINATION | VILLAGE BUILDING | SERVICES | NETWORKING |
|-------------------|---------------|------------------|--------------------|------------------|----------|------------|
| 1.0 | 0 | 6 | 0 | 0 | 6 | 0 |

| STORY ID | CLOGGERS | | MAP | 3 | | DATE(S) | | 5/97 TO 7/97 |
|----------|----------|--|-----|---|--|---------|--|--------------|

| WHO | POP | TYPE | DID WHAT | LEVEL | MULT |
|-----|-----|------|----------|-------|------|
| DIRECTOR | 1 | S | SUPPORTED CLOGGING PROGRAM WITH RESOURCES | ACT3 | 0 |

| FOR WHOM | POP | TYPE | WITH WHAT RESULT | LEVEL | MULT |
|----------|-----|------|------------------|-------|------|
| INSTRUCTORS | 2 | C | ENABLED TO TEACH CLOGGING CLASS | LEV3 | 2 |

| LEVERAGE FRACTION | ACTION POINTS | RECIPIENT POINTS | SELF-DETERMINATION | VILLAGE BUILDING | SERVICES | NETWORKING |
|-------------------|---------------|------------------|--------------------|------------------|----------|------------|
| 1.0 | 0 | 6 | 0 | 0 | 6 | 0 |

| STORY ID | CLOGGERS | | MAP | 4 | | DATE(S) | | 8/97 TO 10/97 |
|----------|----------|--|-----|---|--|---------|--|---------------|

| WHO | POP | TYPE | DID WHAT | LEVEL | MULT |
|-----|-----|------|----------|-------|------|
| DIRECTOR | 1 | S | SUPPORTED CLOGGING PROGRAM WITH RESOURCES | ACT3 | 0 |

| FOR WHOM | POP | TYPE | WITH WHAT RESULT | LEVEL | MULT |
|----------|-----|------|------------------|-------|------|
| INSTRUCTORS | 2 | C | ENABLED TO TEACH CLOGGING CLASS | LEV3 | 2 |

| LEVERAGE FRACTION | ACTION POINTS | RECIPIENT POINTS | SELF-DETERMINATION | VILLAGE BUILDING | SERVICES | NETWORKING |
|-------------------|---------------|------------------|--------------------|------------------|----------|------------|
| 1.0 | 0 | 6 | 0 | 0 | 6 | 0 |

| STORY ID | CLOGGERS | | MAP 5 | DATE(S) 11/97++ | |
|---|---|---|---|---|---|
| WHO | POP | TYPE | DID WHAT | LEVEL | MULT |
| DIRECTOR | 1 | S | SUPPORTED CLOGGING PROGRAM WITH RESOURCES | ACT3 | 0 |
| FOR WHOM | POP | TYPE | WITH WHAT RESULT | LEVEL | MULT |
| INSTRUCTORS | 2 | C | ENABLED TO TEACH CLOGGING CLASS | LEV3 | 2 |

| LEVERAGE FRACTION | ACTION POINTS | RECIPIENT POINTS | SELF-DETERMINATION | VILLAGE BUILDING | SERVICES | NETWORKING |
|---|---|---|---|---|---|---|
| 1.0 | 0 | 6 | 0 | 0 | 6 | 0 |

*Map 6.* Twelve seniors were attracted to the program via the announcement on the bulletin board. The change agent were staff and hence no action points were earned. The recipients were the 12 seniors who saw the notice and signed up (others probably saw the notice as well, but were not counted in this Level 1 transaction, since it did not add anything to their health or well-being—that is, there were no health facts or tips). Thus, the client service points were 1 × 4 = 4 (since the population multiplier for 12 persons is 4).

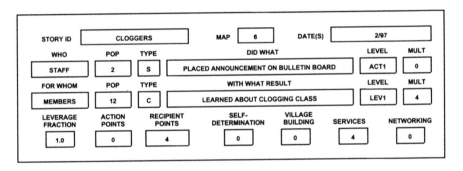

| STORY ID | CLOGGERS | | MAP 6 | DATE(S) 2/97 | |
|---|---|---|---|---|---|
| WHO | POP | TYPE | DID WHAT | LEVEL | MULT |
| STAFF | 2 | S | PLACED ANNOUNCEMENT ON BULLETIN BOARD | ACT1 | 0 |
| FOR WHOM | POP | TYPE | WITH WHAT RESULT | LEVEL | MULT |
| MEMBERS | 12 | C | LEARNED ABOUT CLOGGING CLASS | LEV1 | 4 |

| LEVERAGE FRACTION | ACTION POINTS | RECIPIENT POINTS | SELF-DETERMINATION | VILLAGE BUILDING | SERVICES | NETWORKING |
|---|---|---|---|---|---|---|
| 1.0 | 0 | 4 | 0 | 0 | 4 | 0 |

*Maps 7–10.* The instructors provided clogging instruction for 12 members of the center. The population multiplier of 4 was applied to the results level 3 (ACT3→LEV3) to yield the 12 recipient (and client service) points. The time period was February through November (10 months), resulting in the four maps. The activity did not advance to ACT5→LEV5 after six months, since it was a single service and the instructors continued to be the driving force behind the program (i.e., there was no intention to convert the students to instructors).

| STORY ID | CLOGGERS | | MAP | 7 | DATE(S) | 2/97 TO 4/97 | |
|---|---|---|---|---|---|---|---|

| WHO | POP | TYPE | DID WHAT | LEVEL | MULT |
|---|---|---|---|---|---|
| INSTRUCTORS | 2 | VC | TAUGHT CLOGGING TWICE WEEKLY | ACT3 | 2 |

| FOR WHOM | POP | TYPE | WITH WHAT RESULT | LEVEL | MULT |
|---|---|---|---|---|---|
| MEMBERS | 12 | C | PARTICIPATED IN HEALTHY AND ENJOYABLE ACTIVITY | LEV3 | 4 |

| LEVERAGE FRACTION | ACTION POINTS | RECIPIENT POINTS | SELF-DETERMINATION | VILLAGE BUILDING | SERVICES | NETWORKING |
|---|---|---|---|---|---|---|
| 1.0 | 6 | 12 | 0 | 6 | 12 | 0 |

| STORY ID | CLOGGERS | | MAP | 8 | DATE(S) | 5/97 TO 7/97 | |
|---|---|---|---|---|---|---|---|

| WHO | POP | TYPE | DID WHAT | LEVEL | MULT |
|---|---|---|---|---|---|
| INSTRUCTORS | 2 | VC | TAUGHT CLOGGING TWICE WEEKLY | ACT3 | 2 |

| FOR WHOM | POP | TYPE | WITH WHAT RESULT | LEVEL | MULT |
|---|---|---|---|---|---|
| MEMBERS | 12 | C | PARTICIPATED IN HEALTHY AND ENJOYABLE ACTIVITY | LEV3 | 4 |

| LEVERAGE FRACTION | ACTION POINTS | RECIPIENT POINTS | SELF-DETERMINATION | VILLAGE BUILDING | SERVICES | NETWORKING |
|---|---|---|---|---|---|---|
| 1.0 | 6 | 12 | 0 | 6 | 12 | 0 |

| STORY ID | CLOGGERS | | MAP | 9 | DATE(S) | 8/97 TO 10/97 | |
|---|---|---|---|---|---|---|---|

| WHO | POP | TYPE | DID WHAT | LEVEL | MULT |
|---|---|---|---|---|---|
| INSTRUCTORS | 2 | VC | TAUGHT CLOGGING TWICE WEEKLY | ACT3 | 2 |

| FOR WHOM | POP | TYPE | WITH WHAT RESULT | LEVEL | MULT |
|---|---|---|---|---|---|
| MEMBERS | 12 | C | PARTICIPATED IN HEALTHY AND ENJOYABLE ACTIVITY | LEV3 | 4 |

| LEVERAGE FRACTION | ACTION POINTS | RECIPIENT POINTS | SELF-DETERMINATION | VILLAGE BUILDING | SERVICES | NETWORKING |
|---|---|---|---|---|---|---|
| 1.0 | 6 | 12 | 0 | 6 | 12 | 0 |

| STORY ID | CLOGGERS | | MAP | 10 | DATE(S) | 11/97++ | |
|---|---|---|---|---|---|---|---|

| WHO | POP | TYPE | DID WHAT | LEVEL | MULT |
|---|---|---|---|---|---|
| INSTRUCTORS | 2 | VC | TAUGHT CLOGGING TWICE WEEKLY | ACT3 | 2 |

| FOR WHOM | POP | TYPE | WITH WHAT RESULT | LEVEL | MULT |
|---|---|---|---|---|---|
| MEMBERS | 12 | C | PARTICIPATED IN HEALTHY AND ENJOYABLE ACTIVITY | LEV3 | 4 |

| LEVERAGE FRACTION | ACTION POINTS | RECIPIENT POINTS | SELF-DETERMINATION | VILLAGE BUILDING | SERVICES | NETWORKING |
|---|---|---|---|---|---|---|
| 1.0 | 6 | 12 | 0 | 6 | 12 | 0 |

*Maps 11 and 12.* The group of 14 (two instructors plus 12 class partici-pants, all of whom are clients of the center) performed in nursing homes around the county, reaching over 200 persons. Since this was over a four-month period, it required two maps. The data did not indicate how many of the 200 persons were reached each month, so an equal number per month (50) was assumed. Performances are coded as ACT2→LEV2 (i.e., motivational rather than direct service impact). In Map 11, the action (village building) points were 2 × 2 = 4 (since the 14 change agents functioned as a group, carrying a population value of 2, by convention). The service points (to those entertained) were 2 × 7 = 14 (since 150 persons carries a population multiplier of 7). In Map 12, the village building points were also 2 × 2 = 4. The service points (to those entertained) were 2 × 5 = 10 (since 50 persons carries a population multiplier of 5).

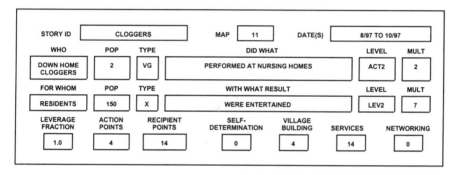

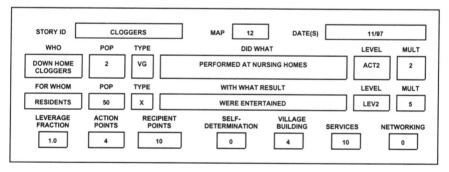

*Maps 13 and 14.* Milestones (MLS4s) were awarded to the two instructors (who also were center members) for organizing and facilitating the class and the outreach to nursing homes. This presumably contributed to their sense of mental health and well-being. Each earned 4 × 1 = 4 action (self-determination) points. A MLS6 did not seem warranted, since this was not a dramatic life style change—and there was no Level 5 activity. The leverage fraction was 1.0, since the two instructors were one step removed from the program staff and supported at Level 3 (documented in Maps 2–5).

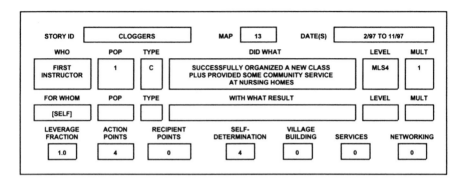

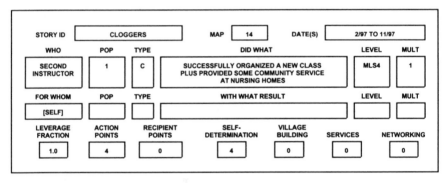

There was not enough information provided in the story to warrant, with certainty, a map with milestones for the 12 student cloggers at either MLS4 or MLS6. In other words, beyond being class members and occasional performers, it is not claimed that they had taken additional actions to increase their health and well-being. However, given their age and their willingness to perform at nursing homes, a milestone (MLS4) for each of the 12 class members might also have been assigned (as Maps 15–26). One such map would have appeared as follows:

| STORY ID | CLOGGERS | | MAP | 18 | DATE(S) | 2/97 TO 11/97 | |
|---|---|---|---|---|---|---|---|

| WHO | POP | TYPE | DID WHAT | LEVEL | MULT |
|---|---|---|---|---|---|
| CLOGGER | 1 | C | EXHIBITED INCREASED HEALTH FROM EXERCISE PLUS ENTERTAINED PEERS AT NURSING HOMES | MLS4 | 1 |

| FOR WHOM | POP | TYPE | WITH WHAT RESULT | LEVEL | MULT |
|---|---|---|---|---|---|
| [SELF] | | | | | |

| LEVERAGE FRACTION | ACTION POINTS | RECIPIENT POINTS | SELF-DETERMINATION | VILLAGE BUILDING | SERVICES | NETWORKING |
|---|---|---|---|---|---|---|
| 1.0 | 4 | 0 | 4 | 0 | 0 | 0 |

We would need more information about the health/wellness status of each of the 12 cloggers, before and during participation, to determine whether these milestones were warranted.

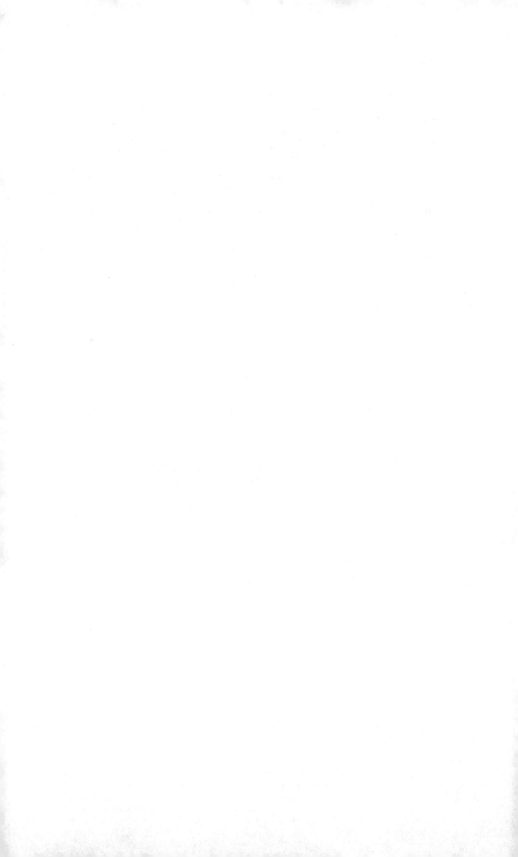

# Appendix B

## Summary of Rules and Conventions

1. Results Mapping is used to map, score, analyze, and provide feedback to improve the best work that a program does with its cl-I-ents.[1] Each story features some of that best work. It is not the cl-I-ent's life story that is being presented. Nor is it only the interface of the program with the cl-I-ent. Rather, it is a story that *begins* with the first interaction between the program and the cl-I-ent and *extends* to further such interactions, to program interactions with the cl-I-ent's support system, to cl-I-ent interchanges with others mobilized by the program to assist the cl-I-ent, *and* to personal cl-I-ent achievements in support of self or to benefit others.
2. Excluded from the story are services provided to the cl-I-ent by other agencies that are not linked to earlier program actions to benefit the cl-I-ent. Also excluded are cl-I-ent activities and achievements that are not linked to the program's objectives *or* are well beyond the contributions of the program to these achievements.
3. Map 1 must be a transactional map with program staff (or volunteer staff) as the change agent.
4. If information relating to the time period before initial staff involvement is pertinent, this information may be presented as Map 0—but is not scored.
5. Maps of a story should be presented in roughly chronological order to capture all significant contributions of the program to current and future successes of the cl-I-ent. These include contributions where program staff are the change agent but also contributions made through the efforts of others that can be linked back to earlier, related program efforts.

[1] As discussed at the start of Chapter 5, cl-I-ent (with a capital "I") is used in the second half of the book to emphasize that the projects being evaluated through Results Mapping work with subjects, not objects, to foster self-determination, growth, health, and emergence of creative potential.

6. Each change agent action that is mapped is coded (with an ACTn or MLSn), as is each recipient response (with a LEVn). For a self-referential map, where there is no recipient, only the change agent action is coded. For a transactional map, the results level (n) is the same for both the ACTn and the LEVn codes.

7. There are seven results levels used to code maps. Three of these levels only are reached on self-referential maps (and are distinguished from the others by changing the ACTn code to a MLSn code—for personal "milestone"). The remaining four levels are reached on both transactional and self-referential maps, although they are far more common in transactional maps.

ACT1/LEV1 Information is obtained without direct interaction with its provider

ACT2/LEV2 Information, brief advice, or some auxiliary service is received through contact with the provider

ACT3/LEV3 A primary service is received through interaction with the provider

MLS4 An adjustment in lifestyle, life status, or program operations is made that is sustained more than one month

ACT5/LEV5 A sustained relationship (more than six months) is maintained with the provider that involves multiple services and is intended to move the cl-I-ent beyond dependency on the provider

MLS6 An adjustment in lifestyle, life status, or program operations is sustained for more than six months *and* concrete gains can be shown that directly relate to these changes

MLS7 The full benefits of changes in lifestyle, life status, or program operations are reaped as reflected in some truly exceptional performance or contribution

8. Staff of the program being evaluated never receive points as recipients of a map of a story. Results Mapping focuses on the role of the program staff in providing services and leveraging the actions of others (through networking) on behalf of the cl-I-ent. Points are awarded for these contributions. Should a staffer obtain some special information, assistance, or training as a prerequisite for further actions in a story, these acquisitions may be noted in the story but are not scored (i.e., they are treated similarly to a background map).

9. Internal handoffs are not mapped. As the story progresses, different program staff may become involved. There is no need to map the "handoff" from one staffer to another. This is assumed and furthermore would not earn the program any additional points. Similarly, once a handoff is

made to another service provider, should there be internal handoffs within the provider agency, these handoffs are not mapped.

10. All change agents of maps of a story need to be linked back to the program being evaluated. A change agent cannot appear in a map of a story until that individual has first appeared in the story as a recipient of an earlier map. Exceptions to this rule are program staff or staff of another entity mobilized by the program that enter the story through internal handoffs. Also excepted are family members of the cl-I-ent, who can be mapped as change agents without showing a handoff from the cl-I-ent to them (viewed as a type of internal handoff).

11. The following codes are used to indicate the type of change agent or recipient:

| | |
|---|---|
| S | Program staff |
| C | Cl-I-ent |
| F | Family member of the cl-I-ent |
| P | Individual provider or professional (not staff) |
| G | Group (team, committee, organization, institution, or system) |
| X | Other community member |

When the change agent performed the action as a volunteer, a "V" is placed before the code. For example, a volunteer organization would be coded as "VG," a doctor providing free medical care would be coded as "VP," and a citizen serving as a volunteer would be coded as "VX."

12. A volunteer from the community who provided a one-time or short-lived service is coded as "VX." However, if the service was ongoing (e.g., serving as a mentor or care giver) and the program being evaluated provided logistical or other support for the volunteer, then the latter is coded as "VS." This has important implications for leveraging. Furthermore, an individual coded with "VS" can kick off a story (as Map 1).

13. Population multipliers are used to account for multiple change agents or multiple recipients in the action being mapped. A quasi-logarithmic scale is used to convert the actual number of change agents or recipients to the corresponding population multiplier.

| Actual number | Population multiplier | Actual number | Population multiplier |
|---|---|---|---|
| 1 | 1 | 51–100 | 6 |
| 2–5 | 2 | 101–500 | 7 |
| 6–10 | 3 | 501–1,000 | 8 |
| 11–25 | 4 | 1,001–10,000 | 9 |
| 26–50 | 5 | 10,001+ | 10 |

14. For transactional maps, when change agents are *not* volunteers (i.e., they are program staff or others being paid to deliver the service), the population multiplier assigned to the *change agent portion* of the map is 0. This insures that village building points are not earned for this activity. As a simple check, if the code for the change agent type begins with a "V" (e.g., VS or VG or VX), then use the conversion table above to determine the population multiplier for the change agents; otherwise, assign a "0" to that value.

15. When the change agent or recipient of a map is a collective (coded as "G"), the *actual population* assigned to that entity is 2, as is the population multiplier. This convention applies to task forces, clinics, coalitions, funding groups, teams, schools, and other aggregates. There are two exceptions, however. First, when this entity is operating as the change agent of a map, if there is no "V" in the code indicating that the entity is serving in a volunteer capacity, the *population multiplier* assigned is "0." Second, when the entity is the recipient of a handoff (rather than being provided with some direct service), the *actual population* assigned to the map is "1," as is the population multiplier.

    *Note:* When a single representative of that organization takes action or receives a service, then the code used is "P" and not "G" and the population value is 1 and not 2.

16. Map leverage fractions are used to account for actions taken by parties other than program staff that may be far removed from the program or that catalyze impacts beyond the results levels for which the program should claim full credit. To determine the fraction, first observe who is the change agent. If the change agent is a program staffer, the fraction is automatically assigned a value of "1." If the change agent is not a program staffer, two tests are used to determine the leverage fraction:

    *First,* how far separated is the change agent from any program staffer in a related map? If there is one degree of separation (i.e., there was direct contact between any staffer and this change agent in some earlier map), the leverage fraction remains at "1." If there are two degrees of separation (i.e., the connection between any staffer and this change agent is through some intermediate change agent), the leverage fraction becomes "0.5" and half credit is earned by the program for the accomplishments on this map. If there are more than two degrees of separation, the leverage fraction becomes "0" and no credit is earned by the program for the accomplishments on this map.

    *Second,* if the leverage fraction is not already "0," compare the results level of the map against the highest results level of a previous related map where a staffer was the change agent. If the results level of the current map is lower, the same as, or one level higher than the level of that staff map, the leverage fraction does not change. If the results level of the current map is two levels higher than the staff map, the leverage fraction remains or is changed to "0.5." If the results level of the current map is three or more levels higher than the staff map, the leverage fraction is changed to "0."

17. The change agent points earned by the program for a map are computed by multiplying the results level on the ACTn/MLSn code (i.e., the "n") by the change agent population multiplier and by the map leverage fraction. The recipient points earned by the program for that map are computed by multiplying the results level on the LEVn code (i.e., the "n") by the recipient population multiplier and by the same leverage fraction.

18. The sum of the change agent points and recipient points is the map score. The sum of the map scores for all the maps of a story is the story score.

19. The map score points are also categorized as follows:

    *Service/networking points:* Points earned by the program on transactional maps for benefits to recipients. When a cl-I-ent is the recipient, these are called cl-I-ent *service* points; when a family member is the recipient, these are called family member *service* points; when a professional is the recipient (e.g., a trainee at a program facilitated by staff), these are called professional *service* points; etc. However, when the recipient points represent a handoff to another entity, these are referred to as *networking* points.

    *Self-determination points:* Points earned by the program for self-referential maps. Usually it is the cl-I-ent of the story who has taken the actions for self-improvement or self-efficacy. However, a family member (for family benefit) or a community group (for future community benefit) might also earn self-determination points.

    *Village-building points:* Points earned by the program for transactional maps, where the change agent is a volunteer. Thus, for example, a doctor who provided charity care would earn the program village-building points when program staff referred a cl-I-ent to that doctor for services. Similarly, a volunteer staffer who served as a mentor for a young child would earn the program village building points.

20. If a change agent provided the same service to a recipient multiple times during the same three-month period using the same basic mode of delivery (e.g., weekly counseling), it is mapped only once. However, if the service continued beyond three months, for each additional three-month segment or less, a new map would be added to the story. Thus, for example, a service that is provided continually for 11 months would result in four maps, one for each three-month period.

21. When services are directed at *different* cl-I-ent objectives, then multiple maps are used. Thus, for example, if a change agent provided services to a recipient aimed at improving the latter's reading skills while also providing services to that recipient dealing with some health issue, each set

of services would be mapped separately. For either set of services, the three-month rule would apply.

22. A level 5 relationship (e.g., mentoring) must be mapped for six months at level 3 before being elevated to level 5. Note: This convention ensures satisfaction of the condition for a level 5 relationship that it be sustained for more than six months. It should be preceded by or associated with a MLS4 map.

23. When the program refers a cl-I-ent or family member to a future change agent (i.e., a handoff), the map showing this referral has the program staff as the map's change agent and the future change agent as its recipient. This holds true even when direct communications between the two did not occur. So, for example, if the program told a cl-I-ent about a provider, and the cl-I-ent made that contact and received the service, the map describing the referral is still shown as a handoff from the program to the provider.

24. For handoffs, the recipient population is always "1."

25. A set of related maps are used to document assisted handoffs. These are cases when either or both of the following situations arise: (a) the cl-I-ent took unusual steps—for him or her—to follow through on the referral with the second agency and/or (b) the program staff provided one or more auxiliary services (e.g., transportation or child care) to allow the cl-I-ent to follow through. Auxiliary services are coded as ACT2/LEV2 and not as ACT3/LEV3, as they would be if primary services. Similarly, the unusual steps taken by the cl-I-ent are coded as ACT2 (self-determination) and not as MLS4.

26. When a map has multiple change agents including both volunteers and non-volunteers, the map is split into two or more maps (since the volunteers earn village building points and the non-volunteers do not). In split maps of this type, the recipient is only listed once to avoid double counting, or a population of 0 is used in the second map. Further, if there are multiple change agents of the same type (e.g., volunteers) but with different associated leverage fractions, then the leverage fraction that would apply to the majority of the group is used to score the map.

27. Similarly, when a map has different types of recipients that the program is interested in tracking separately (e.g., the client versus other family members), then the map is split into two or more maps. In split maps of this type, the change agent is only listed once to avoid double counting of village building points, or a population of 0 is used.

28. When mapping a story, it may be useful to go back more than two years to capture the full extent of program involvement with the cl-I-ent. However, in scoring that story, only maps with dates of two years or less from the cutoff date for the next report are scored. Points for earlier maps are zeroed out.

# Appendix C

## Questionnaire for Compiling Story Data

1. Name of cl-I-ent:
2. Brief description of cl-I-ent:
3. Outcome target(s) of interest:
4. Date, reason for initial program contact, and how initiated:

| Date | Reason | How initiated |
|------|--------|---------------|
|      |        |               |

5. Services provided by staff or volunteer staff during past two years (in 3-month blocks):

| Dates | Services | Purpose | Vol (Y/N)? |
|-------|----------|---------|------------|
|       |          |         |            |
|       |          |         |            |
|       |          |         |            |
|       |          |         |            |
|       |          |         |            |
|       |          |         |            |

6. Handoffs to other providers or support persons during past two years (in three-month blocks):

| Dates | Provider | Services | Purpose | Vol (Y/N)? |
|---|---|---|---|---|
|  |  |  |  |  |
|  |  |  |  |  |
|  |  |  |  |  |
|  |  |  |  |  |

7. Cl-I-ent (or family member) achievements of note (for self-benefit):

| Dates | Achievements |
|---|---|
|  |  |
|  |  |
|  |  |
|  |  |

8. Cl-I-ent (or family member) achievements of note (to benefit others):

| Dates | Achievements | To benefit whom |
|---|---|---|
|  |  |  |
|  |  |  |
|  |  |  |

9. Brief description of current status of cl-I-ent:

# Appendix D

## Blank Mapping Forms[1]

| STORY ID | | | MAP | | DATE(S) | | |
|---|---|---|---|---|---|---|---|
| WHO | POP | TYPE | DID WHAT | | | LEVEL | MULT |
| | | | | | | | |
| FOR WHOM | POP | TYPE | WITH WHAT RESULT | | | LEVEL | MULT |
| | | | | | | | |
| LEVERAGE FRACTION | ACTION POINTS | RECIPIENT POINTS | SELF-DETERMINATION | VILLAGE BUILDING | SERVICES | NETWORKING | |

| STORY ID | | | MAP | | DATE(S) | | |
|---|---|---|---|---|---|---|---|
| WHO | POP | TYPE | DID WHAT | | | LEVEL | MULT |
| | | | | | | | |
| FOR WHOM | POP | TYPE | WITH WHAT RESULT | | | LEVEL | MULT |
| | | | | | | | |
| LEVERAGE FRACTION | ACTION POINTS | RECIPIENT POINTS | SELF-DETERMINATION | VILLAGE BUILDING | SERVICES | NETWORKING | |

[1] Note: Copy more pages as needed to complete the exercises.

| STORY ID | | MAP | | DATE(S) | |
|---|---|---|---|---|---|
| WHO | POP | TYPE | DID WHAT | | LEVEL | MULT |
| | | | | | | |
| FOR WHOM | POP | TYPE | WITH WHAT RESULT | | LEVEL | MULT |
| | | | | | | |
| LEVERAGE FRACTION | ACTION POINTS | RECIPIENT POINTS | SELF-DETERMINATION | VILLAGE BUILDING | SERVICES | NETWORKING |
| | | | | | | |

| STORY ID | | MAP | | DATE(S) | |
|---|---|---|---|---|---|
| WHO | POP | TYPE | DID WHAT | | LEVEL | MULT |
| | | | | | | |
| FOR WHOM | POP | TYPE | WITH WHAT RESULT | | LEVEL | MULT |
| | | | | | | |
| LEVERAGE FRACTION | ACTION POINTS | RECIPIENT POINTS | SELF-DETERMINATION | VILLAGE BUILDING | SERVICES | NETWORKING |
| | | | | | | |

| STORY ID | | MAP | | DATE(S) | |
|---|---|---|---|---|---|
| WHO | POP | TYPE | DID WHAT | | LEVEL | MULT |
| | | | | | | |
| FOR WHOM | POP | TYPE | WITH WHAT RESULT | | LEVEL | MULT |
| | | | | | | |
| LEVERAGE FRACTION | ACTION POINTS | RECIPIENT POINTS | SELF-DETERMINATION | VILLAGE BUILDING | SERVICES | NETWORKING |
| | | | | | | |

| STORY ID | | MAP | | DATE(S) | |
|---|---|---|---|---|---|
| WHO | POP | TYPE | DID WHAT | | LEVEL | MULT |
| | | | | | | |
| FOR WHOM | POP | TYPE | WITH WHAT RESULT | | LEVEL | MULT |
| | | | | | | |
| LEVERAGE FRACTION | ACTION POINTS | RECIPIENT POINTS | SELF-DETERMINATION | VILLAGE BUILDING | SERVICES | NETWORKING |
| | | | | | | |

**Form 1**

STORY ID [          ]    MAP [      ]    DATE(S) [          ]

| WHO | POP | TYPE | DID WHAT | LEVEL | MULT |
|---|---|---|---|---|---|
| [  ] | | [  ] | [                    ] | [  ] | [  ] |

| FOR WHOM | POP | TYPE | WITH WHAT RESULT | LEVEL | MULT |
|---|---|---|---|---|---|
| [  ] | | [  ] | [                    ] | [  ] | [  ] |

| LEVERAGE FRACTION | ACTION POINTS | RECIPIENT POINTS | SELF-DETERMINATION | VILLAGE BUILDING | SERVICES | NETWORKING |
|---|---|---|---|---|---|---|
| [  ] | [  ] | [  ] | [  ] | [  ] | [  ] | [  ] |

**Form 2**

STORY ID [          ]    MAP [      ]    DATE(S) [          ]

| WHO | POP | TYPE | DID WHAT | LEVEL | MULT |
|---|---|---|---|---|---|
| [  ] | | [  ] | [                    ] | [  ] | [  ] |

| FOR WHOM | POP | TYPE | WITH WHAT RESULT | LEVEL | MULT |
|---|---|---|---|---|---|
| [  ] | | [  ] | [                    ] | [  ] | [  ] |

| LEVERAGE FRACTION | ACTION POINTS | RECIPIENT POINTS | SELF-DETERMINATION | VILLAGE BUILDING | SERVICES | NETWORKING |
|---|---|---|---|---|---|---|
| [  ] | [  ] | [  ] | [  ] | [  ] | [  ] | [  ] |

**Form 3**

STORY ID [          ]    MAP [      ]    DATE(S) [          ]

| WHO | POP | TYPE | DID WHAT | LEVEL | MULT |
|---|---|---|---|---|---|
| [  ] | | [  ] | [                    ] | [  ] | [  ] |

| FOR WHOM | POP | TYPE | WITH WHAT RESULT | LEVEL | MULT |
|---|---|---|---|---|---|
| [  ] | | [  ] | [                    ] | [  ] | [  ] |

| LEVERAGE FRACTION | ACTION POINTS | RECIPIENT POINTS | SELF-DETERMINATION | VILLAGE BUILDING | SERVICES | NETWORKING |
|---|---|---|---|---|---|---|
| [  ] | [  ] | [  ] | [  ] | [  ] | [  ] | [  ] |

**Form 4**

STORY ID [          ]    MAP [      ]    DATE(S) [          ]

| WHO | POP | TYPE | DID WHAT | LEVEL | MULT |
|---|---|---|---|---|---|
| [  ] | [  ] | [  ] | [                    ] | [  ] | [  ] |

| FOR WHOM | POP | TYPE | WITH WHAT RESULT | LEVEL | MULT |
|---|---|---|---|---|---|
| [  ] | [  ] | [  ] | [                    ] | [  ] | [  ] |

| LEVERAGE FRACTION | ACTION POINTS | RECIPIENT POINTS | SELF-DETERMINATION | VILLAGE BUILDING | SERVICES | NETWORKING |
|---|---|---|---|---|---|---|
| [  ] | [  ] | [  ] | [  ] | [  ] | [  ] | [  ] |

STORY ID [                    ]     MAP [        ]     DATE(S) [                    ]

| WHO | POP | TYPE | DID WHAT | LEVEL | MULT |
|------|-----|------|----------|-------|------|
| [    ] | [    ] | [    ] | [                    ] | [    ] | [    ] |

| FOR WHOM | POP | TYPE | WITH WHAT RESULT | LEVEL | MULT |
|----------|-----|------|------------------|-------|------|
| [    ] | [    ] | [    ] | [                    ] | [    ] | [    ] |

| LEVERAGE FRACTION | ACTION POINTS | RECIPIENT POINTS | SELF-DETERMINATION | VILLAGE BUILDING | SERVICES | NETWORKING |
|-------------------|---------------|------------------|--------------------|------------------|----------|------------|
| [    ] | [    ] | [    ] | [    ] | [    ] | [    ] | [    ] |

---

STORY ID [                    ]     MAP [        ]     DATE(S) [                    ]

| WHO | POP | TYPE | DID WHAT | LEVEL | MULT |
|------|-----|------|----------|-------|------|
| [    ] | [    ] | [    ] | [                    ] | [    ] | [    ] |

| FOR WHOM | POP | TYPE | WITH WHAT RESULT | LEVEL | MULT |
|----------|-----|------|------------------|-------|------|
| [    ] | [    ] | [    ] | [                    ] | [    ] | [    ] |

| LEVERAGE FRACTION | ACTION POINTS | RECIPIENT POINTS | SELF-DETERMINATION | VILLAGE BUILDING | SERVICES | NETWORKING |
|-------------------|---------------|------------------|--------------------|------------------|----------|------------|
| [    ] | [    ] | [    ] | [    ] | [    ] | [    ] | [    ] |

---

STORY ID [                    ]     MAP [        ]     DATE(S) [                    ]

| WHO | POP | TYPE | DID WHAT | LEVEL | MULT |
|------|-----|------|----------|-------|------|
| [    ] | [    ] | [    ] | [                    ] | [    ] | [    ] |

| FOR WHOM | POP | TYPE | WITH WHAT RESULT | LEVEL | MULT |
|----------|-----|------|------------------|-------|------|
| [    ] | [    ] | [    ] | [                    ] | [    ] | [    ] |

| LEVERAGE FRACTION | ACTION POINTS | RECIPIENT POINTS | SELF-DETERMINATION | VILLAGE BUILDING | SERVICES | NETWORKING |
|-------------------|---------------|------------------|--------------------|------------------|----------|------------|
| [    ] | [    ] | [    ] | [    ] | [    ] | [    ] | [    ] |

---

STORY ID [                    ]     MAP [        ]     DATE(S) [                    ]

| WHO | POP | TYPE | DID WHAT | LEVEL | MULT |
|------|-----|------|----------|-------|------|
| [    ] | [    ] | [    ] | [                    ] | [    ] | [    ] |

| FOR WHOM | POP | TYPE | WITH WHAT RESULT | LEVEL | MULT |
|----------|-----|------|------------------|-------|------|
| [    ] | [    ] | [    ] | [                    ] | [    ] | [    ] |

| LEVERAGE FRACTION | ACTION POINTS | RECIPIENT POINTS | SELF-DETERMINATION | VILLAGE BUILDING | SERVICES | NETWORKING |
|-------------------|---------------|------------------|--------------------|------------------|----------|------------|
| [    ] | [    ] | [    ] | [    ] | [    ] | [    ] | [    ] |

# References

Berne, Eric. (1964). *Games people play: The psychology of human relationships.* New York: Grove Press.

Bohm, David & Peat, F. David. (1987). *Science, order, and creativity.* New York: Bantam Books.

Buber, Martin. (1992). *On intersubjectivity and cultural creativity.* Chicago: The University of Chicago Press. A collection of his writings edited by S. N. Eisenstadt.

Etzioni, Amitai. (1993). *The spirit of community.* New York: Simon and Schuster.

Fetterman, David M., Kaftarian, Shakeh J., & Wandersman, Abraham (Eds.). (1996). *Empowerment evaluation: Knowledge and tools for self-assessment and accountability.* Thousand Oaks, CA: Sage Publications.

Harmon, Willis, & Rheingold, Howard. (1984). *Higher creativity: Liberating the unconscious for breakthrough insights.* Los Angeles: Jeremy P. Tarcher, Inc..

House, E. R. (1994). Integrating the quantitative and qualitative. In C. S. Reichardt and S. F. Rallis (Eds.), *The qualitative-quantitative debate: New perspectives.* New Directions for Program Evaluation, no. 61 (pp.13–22). San Francisco: Jossey-Bass.

Jacobs, Jane. (1961). *The death and life of great American cities.* New York: Random House.

Land, George T. Lock. (1973). *Grow or die: The unifying principle of transformation.* New York: Dell Publishing.

Lofquist, William A. (1989). *The technology of prevention.* Tucson: AYD Publications.

Lofquist, William A. (1996). *The technology of development.* Tucson: Development Publications.

Maslow, Abraham H. (1968). *Toward a psychology of being.* New York: D. Van Nostrand Company.

Morell, Jonathan A. (1979). *Program evaluation in social research.* New York: Pergamon Press.

Osborne, David, & Gaebler, Ted. (1992). *Reinventing government.* New York: Penguin Books.

Peters, Thomas J., & Waterman, Robert H., Jr. (1982). *In search of excellence.* New York: Warner Books.

Scriven, Michael. (1993). *Hard-won lessons in program evaluation.* New Directions for Program Evaluation, no. 58. San Francisco: Jossey-Bass.

Shye, Samuel, Elizur, Dov, & Hoffman, Michael. (1994). *Introduction to facet theory.* Thousand Oaks, CA: Sage Publications.

Stewart, Kathryn, & Klitzner, Michael. (1992). Alcohol and other drug problem prevention from a public health perspective. Background Paper prepared for the Center for Substance Abuse Prevention. Available from the National Center for the Advancement of Prevention, Rockville, MD.

Trochim, William M. K. (Ed.). (1986). *Advances in quasi-experimental design and analysis.* New Directions for Program Evaluation, no. 31. San Francisco: Jossey-Bass.

Waldrop, Mitchell M. (1992). *Complexity*. New York: Simon and Schuster.

Weil, Andrew. (1983). *Health and healing*. Boston: Houghton Mifflin.

Weil, Andrew. (1995). *Spontaneous healing*. New York: Fawcett Columbine.

Weinstein, Neil D., & Sandman, Peter M. (1992). A model of the precaution adoption process. *Health Psychology, 11(3)*, 170–180.

Wheatley, Margaret J., & Kellner-Rogers, Myron. (1996). *A simpler way*. San Francisco: Berrett-Koehler Publishers.

Wilber, Ken, Engler, Jack, & Brown, Daniel P. (1986). *Transformations of consciousness*. Boston: Shambhala.

# Index